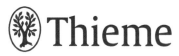

Complications in Non-vascular Interventional Therapy and Interventional Oncology: Cased-based Solutions

Stefan Mueller-Huelsbeck, MD, PhD, EBIR, FICA, FSIR
Professor of Radiology, Board Certified Neuroradiologist
Department of Diagnostic and Interventional Radiology and Neuroradiology
Deaconess Hospital
Flensburg, Germany

Thomas Jahnke, MD, PhD, EBIR, FICA, FSIR
Professor of Radiology
Department of Diagnostic and Interventional Radiology/Nuclear Medicine
Friedrich-Ebert-Hospital
Neumuenster, Germany

With contributions from
Adam Hatzidakis, Afshin Gangi, Alessandro Lunardi, Antonio Basile, Athanasios Pantos,
Attila Kovács, Constantinos T. Sofocleous, Dimitrios Filippiadis, Dimitrios Samonakis,
Douglas Silin, Frédéric Deschamps, Garnon Julien, Georgia Tsoumakidou, Ieva Kurilova,
Ioannis Dedes, Irvin Rexha, Jean Caudrelier, Karin Steinke, Koch Guillaume, Lambros Tselikas,
Laura Crocetti, Milena Miszczuk, Miltiadis E. Krokidis, Nariman Nezami, Nikolaos Galanakis,
Piercarlo Rossi, Rajasekhara R. Ayyagari, Roberto Cioni, Roberto Luigi Cazzato,
Samuel Lewis Rice, Thierry de Baere, Thomas K. Heimberger, Yasuaki Arai

251 illustrations

Thieme
Stuttgart • New York • Delhi • Rio de Janeiro

Library of Congress Cataloging-in-Publication Data

Names: Mueller-Huelsbeck, Stefan, author. | Jahnke, Thomas, author.

Title: Complications in non-vascular interventional therapy and interventional oncology : case-based solutions / Stefan Mueller-Huelsbeck, Thomas Jahnke ; with contributions from Adam Hatzidakis [and others].

Description: Stuttgart ; New York : Thieme, [2019] | Includes bibliographical references and index. | Identifiers: LCCN 2019019129 (print) | LCCN 2019020383 (ebook) | ISBN 9783132413047 () | ISBN 9783132412873 (hardback) | ISBN 9783132413047 (eISBN)

Subjects: | MESH: Radiography, Interventional–adverse effects | Biopsy–adverse effects | Ablation Techniques–adverse effects | Chemoembolization, Therapeutic–adverse effects | Equipment Failure | Case Reports

Classification: LCC RD35 (ebook) | LCC RD35 (print) | NLM WN 202 | DDC 616.07/58–dc23

LC record available at https://lccn.loc.gov/2019019129

© 2019 by Georg Thieme Verlag KG

Thieme Publishers Stuttgart
Rüdigerstrasse 14, 70469 Stuttgart, Germany
+49 [0]711 8931 421, customerservice@thieme.de

Thieme Publishers New York
333 Seventh Avenue, New York, NY 10001 USA
+1 800 782 3488, customerservice@thieme.com

Thieme Publishers Delhi
A-12, Second Floor, Sector-2, Noida-201301
Uttar Pradesh, India
+91 120 45 566 00, customerservice@thieme.in

Thieme Publishers Rio, Thieme Publicações Ltda.
Edifício Rodolpho de Paoli, 25º andar
Av. Nilo Peçanha, 50 – Sala 2508,
Rio de Janeiro 20020-906 Brasil
Tel: +55 21 3172-2297 / +55 21 3172-1896

Cover design: Thieme Publishing Group
Typesetting by Thomson Digital, India

Printed in Germany by CPI Books   5 4 3 2 1

ISBN 978-3-13-241287-3

Also available as an e-book:
eISBN 978-3-13-241304-7

Important note: Medicine is an ever-changing science undergoing continual development. Research and clinical experience are continually expanding our knowledge, in particular our knowledge of proper treatment and drug therapy. Insofar as this book mentions any dosage or application, readers may rest assured that the authors, editors, and publishers have made every effort to ensure that such references are in accordance with **the state of knowledge at the time of production of the book.**

Nevertheless, this does not involve, imply, or express any guarantee or responsibility on the part of the publishers in respect to any dosage instructions and forms of applications stated in the book. **Every user is requested to examine carefully** the manufacturers' leaflets accompanying each drug and to check, if necessary in consultation with a physician or specialist, whether the dosage schedules mentioned therein or the contraindications stated by the manufacturers differ from the statements made in the present book. Such examination is particularly important with drugs that are either rarely used or have been newly released on the market. Every dosage schedule or every form of application used is entirely at the user's own risk and responsibility. The authors and publishers request every user to report to the publishers any discrepancies or inaccuracies noticed. If errors in this work are found after publication, errata will be posted at www.thieme.com on the product description page.

Some of the product names, patents, and registered designs referred to in this book are in fact registered trademarks or proprietary names even though specific reference to this fact is not always made in the text. Therefore, the appearance of a name without designation as proprietary is not to be construed as a representation by the publisher that it is in the public domain.

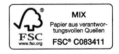

Dedicated to my wife Anke and our children Albert, Viktor, Richard and Felix.

Stefan Mueller-Huelsbeck

Dedicated to my wife Anne and our children Noé and Eliot.

Thomas Jahnke

Contents

Contents

Foreword

Interventional radiologists (IRs) must be aware of the complications of the procedures that they undertake. It is important to note that while all procedures are associated with a list of common complications, some of them may be associated with more esoteric complications, which even though occur rarely, but which IRs should be cognizant of. Every IR should be able to identify the complications and should know the methods of preventing and managing these.

The first step in the management of complications is the knowledge of how to prevent them. Before starting a procedure, the IR should plan each step of the procedure. The old adage "failing to plan means planning to fail" suits best for interventional-radiology procedures. While preparing for a procedure, an IR must consider all the potential complications and plan the procedure around the avoidance of the main complications. Before initiating a procedure an IR should always question "What is the worst thing that can happen in this procedure?" This will help to shift the focus of the IR on avoidance of that complication. For example, when planning to convert a patient with an internal/external biliary drainage catheter to an internal metallic stent, a worst-case scenario in this procedure is losing access when removing the internal/external biliary catheter before inserting the metallic endoprosthesis. If the IR recognizes the potential of this catastrophe, he/she will take extra steps to avoid this situation.

Another important step in the prevention of complications is the use of a safety checklist as described in Chapter 2.[1] The success of a preprocedural checklist before embarking on a procedure is well established and IRs must routinely use a checklist to minimise avoidable complications and mistakes.

The CIRSE classification system was created to provide IRs with a practical method of classifying complications in terms of their severity, management, and implications for any required additional treatment and prolonged hospital stay.[2] IRs should utilise this easy-to-use classification system in their everyday practice.

The editors, Stefan Mueller-Huelsbeck and Thomas Jahnke, have already published a book on complications of vascular interventional radiology procedures. This new book is a companion to the previous book and is focussed on complications of non-vascular and oncological radiological interventions. Both of them are senior interventional radiologists with a worldwide reputation for excellence.

The editors have assembled an outstanding selection of interventional radiologists from around the world who have provided cases that are focussed on various complications. Each case follows a standardised layout and a consistent approach to each complication for the ease of understanding of readers. The cases are divided into categories based on specific type of complications presented. For example, there are sections on bleeding, cement extravasation, and device failure, etc. The cases are beautifully illustrated by images and line drawings to help the reader grasp the concept well.

I would like to congratulate the editors for assembling this magnificent compendium of complications. The book will be of immense value to practising interventional radiologists and trainees.

1. Haynes AB, Weiser TG, Berry WR, et al. Safe Surgery Saves Lives Study Group. A surgical safety checklist to reduce morbidity and mortality in a global population. N Engl J Med. 2009; 360(5): 491–499
2. Filippiadis DK, Binkert C, Pellerin O, Hoffmann RT, Krajina A, Pereira PL. Cirse Quality Assurance Document and Standards for Classification of Complications: The CIRSE Classification System. Cardiovasc Intervent Radiol. 2017; 40 (8):1141–1146

Robert Morgan, MRCP, FRCR, EBIR
President
Cardiovascular and Interventional Radiology Society of Europe (CIRSE);
Consultant Interventional and Diagnostic Radiologist
St George's University Hospitals NHS Foundation Trust
London, UK

Preface

Almost 50 years ago, Charles Dotter performed the first successful angioplasty on an 85-year-old female suffering from gangrene of the forefoot. The procedure was reported successful, resulting in wound healing after minor amputation. Since then, interventional procedures evolved into a widely used approach for treatment of vascular and non-vascular diseases.

Minimally invasive interventional procedures are effective in majority of cases, and are generally characterized by high technical success and low complication rates. However, in case of a few vascular and non-vascular oncologic procedures, adverse events with potentially serious outcomes may occur. In the majority of such cases, complications can be managed by interventional means during or after the initial procedure and are not associated with negative sequelae for the patient. Unfortunately, in some cases, the complications result in serious adverse consequences, causing deterioration of the patients' health for a certain period of time and sometimes even life-long.

In the first edition of our book we focused on vascular interventional complications and their management. In this edition we have provided a review of complications that may occur during *non-vascular* interventional therapy and interventional *oncological* procedures. This edition comprises 45 complication cases that are contributed by renowned specialists in the field. Each case is based on real-life experiences of these specialists and consists of take-home messages for the readers to help them deal with potential problems they may face during their daily interventional practices.

This book will be an invaluable sourcebook for physicians performing non-vascular and oncological interventions. It will aid them to detect as well as avoid and/or manage complications; this book will also help in improving patient care.

The case selection does not claim to be complete in terms of finding the ideal solution to manage a particular problem, however, we hope that the readers will benefit from real-life experiences shared by experienced specialists.

We hope readers will find this compendium an interesting and useful contribution in their daily practice.

Stefan Mueller-Huelsbeck, MD, PhD, EBIR, FICA, FSIR
Thomas Jahnke, MD, PhD, EBIR, FICA, FSIR

Contributors

Adam Hatzidakis, MD, PhD, EBIR
Associate Professor of Radiology
Department of Medical Imaging
University Hospital of Heraklion Crete
Heraklion, Greece

Afshin Gangi, MD, PhD
Professor of Radiology
Department of Interventional Radiology
University Hospital of Strasbourg
Strasbourg, France

Alessandro Lunardi, MD
Interventional Radiologist
Division of Interventional Radiology
University of Pisa
Pisa, Italy

Antonio Basile, MD, EBIR, FCIRSE
Associate Professor of Radiology
Department of Medical Sciences, Surgical,
   and Advanced Technologies
University of Catania
Catania, Italy

Athanasios Pantos, MD, MSc
Interventional Radiologist
Aberdeen Royal Infirmary Hospital
Aberdeen, UK

Attila Kovács, MD
Head of the Clinic
MediClin Robert Janker Clinic
Bonn, Germany

Constantinos T. Sofocleous, MD, PhD
Assistant Professor
Interventional Radiology Service
Memorial Sloan Kettering Cancer Center
New York, NY, USA

Dimitrios Filippiadis, MD, PhD, MSc, EBIR
Assistant Professor of Diagnostic and Interventional
   Radiology
Second Department of Radiology
Medical School, University of Athens
Attikon University Hospital
Athens, Greece

Dimitrios Samonakis, MD
Consultant Gastroenterologist
Department of Gastroenterology
University Hospital of Heraklion Crete
Heraklion, Greece

Douglas Silin, MD
Assistant Professor
Department of Radiology and Biomedical Imaging
   and Department of Vascular and Interventional
   Radiology
Yale School of Medicine
New Haven, CT, USA

Frédéric Deschamps, MD, PHD
Interventional Radiologist
Department of Interventional Radiology
Institut Gustave Roussy
Villejuif, France

Garnon Julien, MD
Associate Professor of Radiology
Department of Interventional Radiology
University Hospital of Strasbourg
Strasbourg, France

Georgia Tsoumakidou, MD
Department of Radiology
University Hospital of Strasbourg
Strasbourg, France

Ieva Kurilova, MD
PhD candidate
Department of Radiology
The Netherlands Cancer Institute
Amsterdam, The Netherlands

Ioannis Dedes, MD
Interventional Oncologist
Department of Diagnostic and Interventional
   Radiology
Interbalkan European Medical Center
Thessaloniki, Greece

Irvin Rexha, MD
Postgraduate Associate
Department of Radiology and Biomedical Imaging
Yale University School of Medicine
Berlin, Germany

Jean Caudrelier, MD, PhD, FRCPC
Radiation Oncologist
Department of Radiation Medicine
The Ottawa Hospital
Ottawa, Canada

Karin Steinke, MD, PhD
Diagnostic/Interventional (non-vascular) Radiologist
Department of Medical Imaging
Royal Brisbane and Women's Hospital
Queensland, Australia

Koch Guillaume, MD
Interventional Radiologist
Department of Interventional Radiology
The University Hospitals of Strasbourg
Strasbourg, France

Lambros Tselikas, MD
Interventional Radiologist
Department of Interventional Radiology
Gustave Roussy
Paris, France

Laura Crocetti, MD, PhD
Professor
Division of Interventional Radiology
University of Pisa
Pisa, Italy

Milena Miszczuk, MD
Junior Doctor
Department of Radiology and Biomedical Imaging
Yale School of Medicine
New Haven, CT, USA

Miltiadis E. Krokidis, MD, PhD, EBIR, FCIRSE, FRCR, FSIR
Consultant Vascular and Interventional Radiologist
Department of Radiology
Cambridge University Hospitals NHS
   Foundation Trust
Cambridge, UK

Nariman Nezami, MD
Resident Diagnostic Radiology
Department of Radiology and Biomedical Imaging
   and Department of Vascular and Interventional
   Radiology
Yale School of Medicine
New Haven, CT, USA

Nikolaos Galanakis, MD
Radiology Resident
Department of Radiology
University Hospital of Heraklion Crete
Heraklion, Greece

Piercarlo Rossi, MD
Interventional Radiologist
Division of Diagnostic and Interventional Radiology
University of Pisa
Pisa, Italy

Rajasekhara R. Ayyagari, MD
Assistant Professor
Department of Radiology and Biomedical Imaging and
   Department of Vascular and Interventional
   Radiology
Yale School of Medicine
New Haven, CT, USA

Roberto Cioni, MD
Interventional Radiologist
Division of Interventional Radiology
University of Pisa
Pisa, Italy

Roberto Luigi Cazzato, MD, PhD
Associate Professor of Radiology
Department of Interventional Radiology
University Hospital of Strasbourg
Strasbourg, France

Samuel Lewis Rice, MD
Assistant Attending of Diagnostic and Interventional
   Radiology
Department of Radiology
Netherlands Cancer Institute
Amsterdam, The Netherlands

Stefan Mueller-Huelsbeck, MD, PhD, EBIR, FICA, FSIR
Professor of Radiology, Board Certified
  Neuroradiologist
Department of Diagnostic and Interventional
  Radiology and Neuroradiology
Diakonissen Hospital Flensburg
Flensburg, Germany

Thierry de Baere, MD
Department of Interventional Radiology
Faculty of Medicine, Paris-Sud University
Paris, France

Thomas K. Heimberger, MD
Professor
Department of diagnostic and interventional
  radiology and nuclear medicine
Hospital of the Technical University of Munich
Munich, Germany

Thomas Jahnke, MD, PhD, EBIR, FICA, FSIR
Professor of Radiology
Department of Diagnostic and Interventional
  Radiology and Nuclear Medicine
Friedrich-Ebert-Hospital Neumuenster
Neumuenster, Germany

Yasuaki Arai, MD, FSIR, FCIRSE
Executive Advisor to President, National
  Cancer Center
Department of Diagnostic Radiology
National Cancer Center Hospital
Tokyo, Japan

1 Introduction

Non-vascular and oncologic interventional procedures are increasingly performed worldwide. They are mainly carried out by interventional radiologists and almost all interventional radiology (IR) units impart these services since they are minimally invasive and provide the opportunity to gain excellent therapeutic options for the patient, thereby increasing quality of life, and overall survival. The first step of IR is often percutaneous liver biopsy, which is the minimally invasive gold standard for the histopathological evaluation of liver lesions. If the suspected diagnosis is proven by the pathologist, percutaneous thermal ablation procedures are preferred for patients who are not amenable to classical surgery. These minimal invasive options are performed with the help of regional or general anaesthesia and they have revolutionized local tumor destruction. Ablative therapies offer multiple advantages—they have no specificity for selected tumor cells, they are tissue-saving, and they show a reduced rate of morbidity and mortality both in young and elderly patients; they can be performed in conjunction with other cancer treatments and may be repeated if necessary; they require mostly only conscious sedation and local anesthesia, and last but not the least, they go along with shorter hospital stay. In liver lesions with typical imaging features for malignancy, biopsy and ablation can be performed in one intervention in order to minimize trauma. In these cases a coaxial system with the possibility to perform biopsy and ablation successively is preferred.

In specific case, for example for patient with oligometastatic pulmonary secondary malignancies, surgical resection is considered potentially curative and has shown evidence to improve survival. However, frequent surgery is not feasible either due to medical and technical reasons or it is refused by the patient. In these cases, minimally invasive therapies have attained increasing utilization, especially thermoablative techniques like radiofrequency and microwave ablation. Thermal ablation techniques are limited to lesions that are not larger than 5 cm in diameter, and success can be impaired by heat deflection in the vicinity of

the vessels. Percutaneous computed tomography–guided interstitial high-dose-rate brachytherapy (iHDR BT) enables the highly conformal administration of therapeutic radiation doses to a circumscribed volume. iHDR BT utilizes a fundamentally different technology from thermal ablation and due to this reason it is independent from the above-mentioned limitations. Moreover, the dose decreases rapidly outside the target volume so that the surrounding healthy tissues can be protected. Because the aim of iHDR BT is not to destroy the target tissue during the intervention, but to induce tissue necrosis developing during approximately 6 weeks in the postinterventional phase, the risk potential of this intervention is comparable to a biopsy procedure. However, every percutaneous manipulation in the lung carries the risk of pneumothorax (3.1% in biopsy). IR can also provide other services in addition to treating local tumors, for example, with the help of local tumor ablation techniques.

Kyphoplasty is a different approach to treat a patient; Balloon kyphoplasty (BK) is effective for the therapy of vertebral compression fractures (VCF) in terms of immediate pain relief, decreased need for painkiller medications, quick functional recovery, and increased mobility. In case of elderly osteoporotic patients who are not amenable for surgery, the pain leads to immobilization, hospitalization, and adjunctive secondary complications. BK is an alternative to conservative medical therapy as well as to stabilizing spine surgery, enabling rapid patient mobilization and prompt reintegration into the social environment. Pain reduction is more pronounced in BK (92%) as compared to vertebroplasty (87%). This might be attributed to the restoration of the collapsed kyphotic angle in BK. The most frequent complication following vertebroplasty and BK is fracture of the adjacent level (41% in vertebroplasty and 30% in BK). This is associated with cement endplate extravasation isolated to the anterior third of the vertebral body.

The examples provided above reflect only some facettes of non-vascular and oncologic services of IR. Due to recent developments in this field, there is a demand for more information about these procedures. This book tries to provide further information on potential and most frequent complications of the procedures in terms of indications and limitations. Reporting procedural complications and discussing their treatment options as well as potential strategies to avoid them will not only enrich the armamentarium of the readers but also help them avoid complications in the first place and to react better in case they occur.

Thomas Edison once said, "Experience is merely the sum of all our mistakes." To some extent this holds true for physicians. In medicine, however, we should rather be able to learn from mistakes that others have made in order to keep harm from our own patients.

2 Minor and Major Complications

2.1 Definition and Reporting System of Complications

Interventional radiology (IR) provides a wide variety of vascular, non-vascular, musculoskeletal, and oncologic minimally invasive techniques that are aimed at therapy or palliation of a broad spectrum of pathological conditions. Outcome data for these techniques are globally evaluated by hospitals, insurance companies, and government agencies targeting a high-quality health care policy, including reimbursement strategies. To analyze effectively the outcome of a technique, accurate reporting of complications is necessary. Throughout the literature, numerous classification systems for grading complications have been reported. Until now, there has been no method for uniform reporting of complications both in terms of definition and grading. In 2017 a document was developed by CIRSE called the CIRSE guideline with an aim to a classification system of complications based on combining outcome and severity of sequelae. CIRSE also developed a patient safety checklist, the use of which is of paramount importance. Using the CIRSE patient safety checklist to ensure practice of homogeneity among different individuals and departments is essential in all IR procedures. In a similar way, reviewing and grading complications should be performed in terms of a uniform and accurate reproducible and validated categorization system.

Only by using a safety checklist, there is a 36% decrease of major complications and postsurgical mortality rates. The Society of Interventional Radiology distinguishes minor and major complications. The definitions of these complications are as follows:

Minor complication: Treatment-related adverse event requiring nominal therapy or no treatment with or without overnight hospitalization for observation.
- No therapy, no consequence.
- Nominal therapy, no consequence; includes overnight admission for observation only.

Major complication: Treatment-related adverse event requiring further therapy with increase in the level of care or prolonged hospitalization.
- Require therapy, minor hospitalization (<48 hours).
- Require major therapy, unplanned increase in level of care, prolonged hospitalization (>48 hours).
- Have permanent adverse sequelae.
- Result in death.

The CIRSE classification system for complications is defined as follows:

Grade 1: Complication during the procedure that could be solved within the same session; no additional therapy, no postprocedure sequelae, no deviation from the normal post-therapeutic course.

Grade 2: Prolonged observation including overnight stay (as a deviation from the normal post-therapeutic course <48 hours); no additional postprocedure therapy, no postprocedure sequelae.

Grade 3: Additional postprocedure therapy or prolonged hospital stay (>48 hours) required; no postprocedure sequelae.

Grade 4: Complication causing permanent mild sequelae (resuming work and independent living).

Grade 5: Complication causing permanent severe sequelae (requiring ongoing assistance in daily life).

Grade 6: Death.

The main aspect for consideration is that a complication that can be treated during the same procedure should be stated as minor complication (grade 1), emphasizing the importance of complications' management through interventionalists.

Further Reading

Filippiadis DK, Binkert C, Pellerin O, Hoffmann RT, Krajina A, Pereira PL. CIRSE Quality Assurance Document and Standards for Classification of Complications: The CIRSE Classification System. Cardiovasc Intervent Radiol. 2017; 40(8):1141–1146

Omary RA, Bettmann MA, Cardella JF, et al. Society of Interventional Radiology Standards of Practice Committee. Quality improvement guidelines for the reporting and archiving of interventional radiology procedures. J Vasc Interv Radiol. 2003; 14(9 Pt 2):S293–S295

Haynes AB, Weiser TG, Berry WR, et al. Safe Surgery Saves Lives Study Group. A surgical safety checklist to reduce morbidity and mortality in a global population. N Engl J Med. 2009; 360(5): 491–499

2.2 Avoiding Complications

Avoiding intervention confusion is concerned with special kinds of complications during interventional therapy: interventional therapy on the wrong body part, performing inadequate procedures, or engaging the wrong person. Engagement confusion is rare with regard to all performed procedures. When it occurs, however, the impact on the patient and the persons involved in the care process is momentous. Intervention confusion is generally considered preventable.

Therefore, the aim of the standard operating procedure (SOP) is to prevent confusion by effective implementation and consistent application of the following three complementary process steps while preparing each patient for endovascular interventions:

1. Preoperative verification process.
2. Marking the engagement location.
3. "Team-time-out" immediately before the start of the intervention.

To achieve success, it is important that all members of the pre- and perioperative teams are actively involved in the process and they effectively communicate with each other.

A patient safety checklist, knowledge of how to deal with impaired renal function, and allergic reaction to contrast media will help to minimize and avoid complications.

2.2.1 Patient Safety

"A good physician treats the disease. A great physician treats the patient who has the disease."

—Sir William Osler.

This citation reflects the importance of taking the patient's condition and existing comorbidities into account.

The aviation industry introduced safety checks before flying because of the many technical considerations that influence the safety of flight and the inability of the human mind to remember all the complex factors that require checking before flying. Air safety is such that there is a 1 in 3

million chance of an accident occurring in an airplane, as opposed to a 1 in 300 chance of an accident happening in a hospital. In 2009, Haynes et al published a surgical safety checklist in the New England Journal of Medicine, which was tested in eight centers worldwide. The use of the checklist resulted in a 36% decrease in postoperative complications and a 36% decrease in mortality after surgery. Use of surgical safety checklists have now become a standard practice throughout the world.

2.2.2 Patient Safety Checklist

Preparation of the patient according to the "CIRSE IR Patient Safety Checklist" is strictly recommended (▶ Fig. 2.1). These essential points will minimize communication and malinformation problems or any further confusion before starting the procedure. The CIRSE checklist might be adapted for dedicated, individual hospital-specific needs.

In addition, the following topics should be recognized:

1. Questions an interventional radiologist should ask before accepting procedures:
   - Is the procedure necessary?
   - Is the patient suitable for the procedure?
   - Will it help the patient?
   - What is the potential for harm?
   - Are there better alternatives?
   - If the IR procedure is not performed, will the patient suffer harm?
2. Items that can influence the competence or performance continuum:
   - Define the scope of IR practice by local hospital conditions, support services and current experience.
   - Consult with peers in regard to complex cases.
   - Recognize when further investigation or observation is necessary.
   - Know your limitations and call for help when required.
   - Refer patients with complex problems beyond your experience to expert centers.
   - Participate in audit and risk management.
   - Participate in analysis of adverse events.

Patient Name	
Patient ID	
Date of Birth	
Male ●	Female ●
Ward	
Referring Physician	

DIAKO IR Patient Safety Checklist*

Procedure:

Date:

DIAKO

PROCEDURE PLANNING	YES	NO	N/A
Discussed referring physician/MDT	☐	☐	☐
Imaging SSS reviewed	☐	☐	☐
Relevant medical history	☐	☐	☐
Informed consent	☐	☐	
CIN prophylaxis	☐	☐	☐
Specific tools present/ordered	☐	☐	☐
Fasting order given	☐	☐	☐
Relevant lab tests ordered	☐	☐	☐
Anaesthesiologist necessary	☐	☐	☐
Anticoagulant medication stopped	☐	☐	☐
Postinterventional (ICU) bed required	☐	☐	☐
Contrast allergy prophylaxis necessary	☐	☐	☐

SIGN IN	YES	NO	N/A
All team members introduced	☐	☐	
All Records with patient	☐	☐	☐
Correct patient/side/site	☐	☐	
Patient fasting	☐	☐	☐
IV access	☐	☐	☐
Monitoring equipment attached	☐	☐	☐
Weight (kg)	☐	☐	☐
Coagulation screen/lab tests checked	☐	☐	☐
Allergies and/or phrophylaxis checked	☐	☐	
Antibiotics/other drugs administered	☐	☐	☐
Consent/complications discussed	☐	☐	

SIGN OUT	YES	NO	N/A
Post-op note written	☐	☐	
Vital signs normal during procedure	☐	☐	☐
Medication and CM recorded	☐	☐	☐
Lab tests ordered	☐	☐	☐
All samples labeled and sent to lab	☐	☐	☐
Procedure results discussed with patient	☐	☐	☐
Post-discharge instruction given	☐	☐	☐
Follow-up tests/imaging ordered	☐	☐	☐
Follow-up OPD appointment made	☐	☐	☐
Procedure results communicated to referrer	☐	☐	

Name: _____ Name: _____ Name: _____

Signature: _____ Signature: _____ Signature: _____

* Modified from RADPASS & WHO SURGICAL CHECKLIST

Fig. 2.1 CIRSE IR Patient Safety Checklist. CIN, contrast-induced neuropathy; CM, contrast media; ICU, Intensive Care Unit; MDT, multidisciplinary team; OPD, Outpatient Department. Reproduced with permission from CIRSE.

3. Steps to prevent harm:
   - Use a safety checklist.
   - Mark the operative site.
   - Involve the patient in the decision-making process (informed consent).
   - Make arrangements for appropriate proctoring for new procedures and technology.
   - Reduce distractions from pagers and telephone calls in the laboratory.
   - Maintain a distraction-free environment for everyone.
   - Know your limitations in terms of individual and system limitations.

2.2.3 Periprocedural Documentation

It is of utmost importance to document and store all the steps of the procedure. Store and later archive fluoroscopic images from time to time, especially when they indicate a significant contribution in the progress of the procedure. While doing that, the operator has the possibility to highlight these steps in the report after storing them in the picture archiving and communication system (PACS).

Further Reading

Cardiovascular and Interventional Radiological Society of Europe (CIRSE). Website: http://www.cirse.org. Accessed May 13, 2019

Lee MJ, Fanelli F, Haage P, Hausegger K, Van Lienden KP. Patient safety in interventional radiology: a CIRSE IR checklist. Cardiovasc Intervent Radiol. 2012; 35(2):244–246

Durack JC. The value proposition of structured reporting in interventional radiology. AJR Am J Roentgenol. 2014; 203(4):734–738

Omary RA, Bettmann MA, Cardella JF, et al. Quality improvement guidelines for the reporting and archiving of interventional radiology procedures. J Vasc Interv Radiol. 2002; 13(9 Pt 1): 879–881

Haynes AB, Weiser TG, Berry WR, et al. Safe Surgery Saves Lives Study Group. A surgical safety checklist to reduce morbidity and mortality in a global population. N Engl J Med. 2009; 360(5): 491–499

2.3 General Complications Related to Non-vascular and Oncologic Procedures

2.3.1 Impaired Renal Function

In case of impaired renal function, patients should be treated according to the current European Society of Urogenital Radiology (ESUR) guidelines. Following these guidelines will minimize problems related to uncontrolled iodized contrast media application. In addition to this, following these recommendations is necessary when any iodinated contrast media application is warranted such as contrast-enhanced computed tomography (CT) scans for lesion detection.

Further Reading

European Society of Urogenital Radiology (ESUR). Website: http://www.esur.org. Accessed May 13, 2019

Stacul F, van der Molen AJ, Reimer P, et al. Contrast Media Safety Committee of European Society of Urogenital Radiology (ESUR). Contrast induced nephropathy: updated ESUR Contrast Media Safety Committee guidelines. Eur Radiol. 2011; 21(12):2527–2541

2.4 Known Allergic Reactions to Contrast Material

Patients with known allergic reactions to contrast material should be prepared according to international guidelines. American College of Radiology (ACR) Manual on Contrast Media, Version 9, 2013 from the ACR Committee on Drugs and Contrast Media will help both preventing and treating acute reactions to contrast media.

Further Reading

American College of Radiology (ACR). Website: http://www.acr.org. Accessed May 13, 2019

Bush WH Jr. Treatment of acute contrast reactions. In: Bush WH Jr, Krecke KN, King BF Jr, Bettmann MA, eds. Radiology Life Support (RAD-LS). London/New York: Arnold/Oxford University Press; 1999:31–51

2.5 Radiation Exposure

Wearing all available protective garments (vest, apron, thyroid protection, and lead glasses) is the most obvious measure. In this context, personalized, optimally fitting lead vests and aprons are essential; radiation protective clothes that are too small, result in an increase of radiation dose to the shoulders, chest, and groin. Loose protective clothing also results in an increase in radiation dose due to gaps, for example, under the armpits. Additionally, badly fitting radiation protection clothing may lead to a decrease in acceptance of protective garments by medical staff. Providing medical staff with their own, personalized lead aprons can increase both acceptance and care-taking of the individualized garment. In this context, custom-built, fancy-colored lead aprons with a name badge could be helpful. Eye protection was the aim of recent recommendations. Lead glasses help to protect eyes of the practitioner. The eyeglasses are also available as optically corrected glasses, which help in keeping unnecessary extra weight off the head.

Also, it is suggested for the radiologist to be familiar with dose management during endovascular therapy in order to avoid radiation exposure for both the patient and the staff; plan the procedure with noninvasive imaging tools such as ultrasound or magnetic resonance imaging (MRI); evaluate existing imaging carefully in order to plan access routes and identify potential risk (bowel, vessel, air space, …); and have strategies for preventing complications.

Functions like "last-image hold," the reference-image function, and simulated road mapping allow the operator to reduce the time of imaging. Simply reducing the pulse rate from continuous imaging to 7.5 images per second results in a 90% dose reduction.

With respect to the inverse square law, the medical staff has to be aware of the position of the X-ray and scatter radiation source and main direction of scatter radiation. Usually, the source of scatter radiation is the patient. Highest levels of scatter radiation are commonly just at the side of the X-ray source. If possible, any angulation of the X-ray source should be on the opposite side of the medical staff, and the medical staff should position themselves at a distance to the source of scatter radiation. Keeping the table at a low position and the detector close to the region of interest also allows the interventional radiologist to maintain a distance from the source of scatter radiation (the patient). Arranging the screen in a position that allows the operator to take a relaxed and physiological position is important. However, in this context again, the position of the operator is important, as a good view on screen might make the operator turn sideway in regard to the main source of scatter radiation, while state-of-the-art radiation protection clothing is often double layered on the front (2×0.25 mm lead equivalent), it is only single-layered on the side and back to keep its weight low. Turning sideway thus leaves less protected body areas exposed. This is also important for the medical staff handling material or taking care of the patient; moving within the interventional suite may result in staff turning their backs toward the X-ray source—keeping distance is most important in such cases.

Interventional radiologist should enhance C-arm–related dose management tools and skills by using additional lead glasses and lead curtains to obtain optimal radiation protection according to the ALARA principle (to keep radiation exposure "as low as reasonably achievable"). Finally, use, if available, needle guidance tools.

Dose management before, during, and after the procedure is of utmost importance to avoid both radiation-induced tissue and skin injuries.

Radiation-induced tissue injuries: Radiation-induced tissue injuries were previously labeled as deterministic effects of radiation. The most important tissue injuries affect the skin and the eye lens. Typically, radiation-induced skin injuries occur after a time delay of days, sometimes weeks following a procedure, in which a threshold of skin exposure has been exceeded. Moreover, the patients are more frequently obese, and obesity is a significant contributing factor to higher exposure. In addition, patients undergoing several interventional procedures in their lifetime are more frequently encountered. Patients at risk for tissue injuries are typically of older age (55–85 years) and suffering from chronic diseases—consequentially requiring multiple imaging and interventional procedures.

Radiation-induced skin injuries: Radiation-induced ulcers are currently reported in less than 1% of all patients undergoing cardiac interventions. Skin reactions related to radiation exposure can be distinguished as either prompt/acute/subacute (from 24 hours up to 2 months) or chronic (> 2 months up to years). Prompt radiation-induced skin reactions occur within less than 2 weeks. The most common prompt skin reaction is an erythematous reaction, which can occur from a few

hours up to 24 hours after exposure of more than 2 Gy. This complication is rarely reported in specialist literature but actually quite commonly observed after long and complex interventional procedures. Acute radiation injury of the skin is characterized by erythema with vesicles, erosion, temporary epilation, and pain and itching persisting up to 9 weeks. Chronic radiation injury of the skin (CRIS) presents with an insidious and variable onset of symptoms ranging from erythema, atrophy, epilation, telangiectasia, and pruritus, as well as pain due to dermal necrosis and ulceration. This occurs typically months to years after several high-dose radiation exposures or a single very high radiation exposure with a cumulative peak skin dose threshold of 10 Gy. Clinically, the typical patient with chronic radiation injury presents with permanent erythema, dermal atrophy, and ulceration.

However, even a lower radiation dose due to an increased radiosensitivity is known for obesity, diabetes, nicotine abuse, previous radiation exposure in the same body region, compromised skin integrity, Fitzpatrick skin types I and II (fair skin), diabetes, autoimmune or connective tissue disease (e.g., scleroderma, lupus erythematosus, and mixed connective tissue disease), hyperthyroidism, and certain drugs. This demonstrates once again that dose management and awareness for radiation safety issues are warranted.

Further Reading

Rehani MM, Gupta R, Bartling S, et al. ICRP. Radiological Protection in Cone Beam Computed Tomography (CBCT). ICRP Publication 129. Ann ICRP. 2015; 44(1):9–127

Hertault A, Maurel B, Midulla M, et al. Editor's choice—minimizing radiation exposure during endovascular procedures: basic knowledge, literature review, and reporting standards. Eur J Vasc Endovasc Surg. 2015; 50(1):21–36

Rathmann N, Haeusler U, Diezler P, et al. Evaluation of radiation exposure of medical staff during CT-guided interventions. J Am Coll Radiol. 2015; 12(1):82–89

Rathmann N, Kostrzewa M, Kara K, et al. Radiation exposure of the interventional radiologist during percutaneous biopsy using a multiaxis interventional C-arm CT system with 3D laser guidance: a phantom study. Br J Radiol. 2015; 88(1055): 20150151

Finch W, Shamsa K, Lee MS. Cardiovascular complications of radiation exposure. Rev Cardiovasc Med. 2014; 15(3):232–244

Ketteler ER, Brown KR. Radiation exposure in endovascular procedures. J Vasc Surg. 2011; 53(1) Suppl:35S–38S

Jaschke W, Schmuth M, Trianni A, Bartal G. Radiation-induced skin injuries to patients: what the interventional radiologist needs to know. Cardiovasc Intervent Radiol. 2017; 40(8): 1131–1140

2.6 Infection

Strategies for preventing infections during endo-vascular procedures include general, preoperative, and operative regimes. These are important because diseased patients are prone to infection (i.e., diabetes, chronic wounds, renal impairment, and malignancies responsible for an impaired immunity).

Further Reading

Society of Interventional Radiology (SIR). Website: http://www.sir-web.org. Accessed May 13, 2019

Reddy P, Liebovitz D, Chrisman H, Nemcek AA, Jr, Noskin GA. Infection control practices among interventional radiologists: results of an online survey. J Vasc Interv Radiol. 2009; 20(8):1070–1074.e5

2.7 Management of Complications

Major periprocedural complications are uncommon in interventions, but they may manifest suddenly and can require swift and orderly response. Although the experience of the surgeon, nursing, and technical staff is important, the relative rarity of serious events makes the use of a checklist a valuable practice, helping to ensure orderly implementation of a preplanned response.

"Planning for failure" is a strategy used by good teams that perform procedures with significant risks. The following comments and examples are mainly related to vascular procedures. However, the knowledge of ways to deal with the problems encountered when performing non-vascular procedures is also essential, for example, to avoid bleeding which might occur during the procedure and to treat bleeding, if occured. Patel et al reported improved endovascular outcomes with a preprocedural "mental rehearsal" in hybrid aortic cases. In 2013, Chen developed a checklist for response to a cerebral artery aneurysm perforation and a separate checklist for thrombosis in neurosurgical interventions. The listed expected responses are from the surgeon, anesthesiologist, nursing, and technologist staff, each with specific roles and responsibilities.

For thrombosis, the interventionist should record the ACT and request an empiric bolus of heparin based on the patient's weight and predetermined dose. If vasospasm is detected at the sheath, intra-arterial nitroglycerin should be given. The nursing

staff should administer fluids, and the technologist should prepare aspiration or thrombolytic devices.

For bleeding complications, the interventionist should clearly communicate to the staff about the complications and plans for correction. Serious bleeding from a superficial femoral artery (SFA) intervention is rare, but a high puncture or concomitant iliac artery intervention can lead to rapid blood loss into the pelvis. A retroperitoneal hemorrhage can quickly result in shock. Clearly and succinctly articulating the problem and the anticipated next steps is critical, and it is important to verbally confirm that team members have heard and understood what was said.

Arterial access should be maintained. Required equipment, such as a covered stent, tourniquet, or occlusion balloon, should be requested. The nurse should maintain fluids and blood products as necessary and request an anesthesiologist to assist if the patient is in extremis. The technologist should alert the operating room staff of the potential need for open conversion, and the operating room should be prepared if endovascular solutions are limited or if there is hemodynamic instability.

2.7.1 Arterial Hemorrhage

Recognition: Team member recognizing abnormal bleeding by hemodynamic instability verbally states the problem, calls for help if needed, ensures that hemodynamic monitors are attached and functional, and evaluate access site or site of suspected vascular injury, if accessible.

Hemorrhage control: Apply manual direct pressure if bleeding is from an accessible, compressible site; maintain access, but consider exchanging for a larger-diameter sheath if needed; perform angiography to confirm cessation of bleeding.

Resuscitation: Large-bore intravenous line, consider more than one, with crystalloid solution (saline or Plasmalyte); notify blood bank, send blood specimen, and request for transfusion; consider reversal of anticoagulation (protamine 1 mg to reverse 100 units of heparin); notify vascular surgeon if endovascular therapy is not practical or if the patient is unstable; notify the operating room staff.

Treatment: Prolonged balloon occlusion, covered stent, coiling, particles, gel foam, and glue injection, external compression, reversal of anticoagulation, surgical treatment including vessel repair and fasciotomy for suspected compartment syndrome.

Communication: Inform accompanying family members of the situation and plans.

2.7.2 Preventing Arterial Hemorrhage

Control carefully the coagulation status before starting the procedure, and check ACT during the procedure.

2.7.3 Device Malfunction

Recognize the instructions for use, read them, and ask for training possibilities for complex devices. Taking proctoring services as well as attending workshops related to the device will help the radiologist to familiarize with the dedicated device technique.

2.7.4 Preventing Device Malfunction

Follow the instructions for use carefully. Have a device specialist and/or a proctor available, when starting new procedures.

Further Reading

Cardiovascular and Interventional Radiological Society of Europe (CIRSE). Website: http://www.cirse.org. Accessed May 13, 2019

Sheth RA, Koottappillil B, Kambadakone A, Ganguli S, Thabet A, Mueller PR. A Quality Improvement Initiative to Reduce Catheter Exchange Rates for Fluoroscopically Guided Gastrostomy Tubes. J Vasc Interv Radiol. 2016 Feb;27(2):251–9.

Skonieczki BD, Wells C, Wasser EJ, Dupuy DE. Radiofrequency and microwave tumor ablation in patients with implanted cardiac devices: is it safe? Eur J Radiol. 2011 Sep;79(3):343–6.

Ferral H, Garza-Berlanga AE, Patel NH. Complications of nonvascular interventions and their management: case-based review. AJR Am J Roentgenol. 2009 Jun;192(6 Suppl):S63–77

Wu CC, Maher MM, Shepard JA. Complications of CT-guided percutaneous needle biopsy of the chest: prevention and management. AJR Am J Roentgenol. 2011 Jun;196(6):W678–82

3 Case-Based Procedure-Related Complications

3.1 Bleeding

3.1.1 Bleeding after Percutaneous Biopsy of Liver Tumor

Patient History

A 70-year-old male with multiple liver tumors suspected hepatocellular carcinoma and portal vein tumor thrombus (▶ Fig. 3.1) received percutaneous needle biopsy to perform genomic analysis of the tumor. He had a medical history of alcoholic hepatitis and diabetes mellitus, but it was well controlled with medication. No coagulopathy was observed.

Initial Treatment

With ultrasonography guidance, two times of percutaneous tumor biopsies through normal liver parenchyma were performed by a hepatobiliary medical oncologist with an 18G Sonopsy needle (Hakko, Tokyo, Japan). A guiding needle was not used.

Problems Encountered during the Treatment

No problems during the procedure were noted.

Imaging Plan

So far no further imaging was planned.

Resulting Complication

Two hours after the biopsy, the patient showed hemorrhagic shock. The emergent contrast-enhanced CT examination revealed bloody ascites and extravasation in the arterial phase (▶ Fig. 3.2).

No finding of extravasation was observed on hepatic arterial digital subtraction angiographies (DSAs) at 2 hours after the biopsy. However, CT

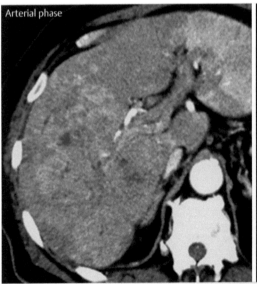
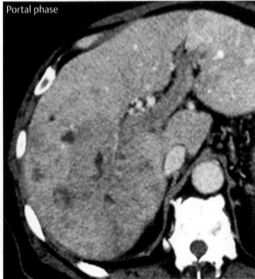

Fig. 3.1 Contrast-enhanced CT shows multiple hypervascular tumors with portal vein tumor thrombus.

during hepatic arteriography via the posterior segmental artery showed significant extravasation (▶ Fig. 3.3); therefore, the posterior branch of the right hepatic artery was embolized with 12.5% glue (NBCA:Lipiodol = 1:7). The second angiography was performed 5 hours after the biopsy because of unstable vital signs, and the additional embolization of A6 was carried out without

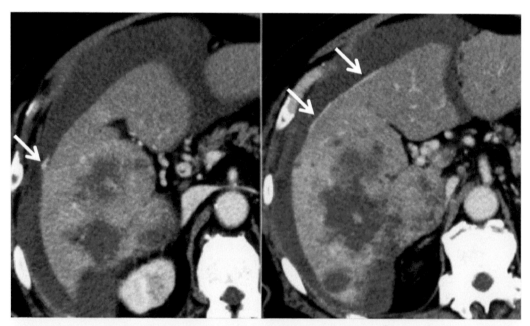

Fig. 3.2 Contrast-enhanced CT shows extravasation of contrast at the liver surface (*arrows*).

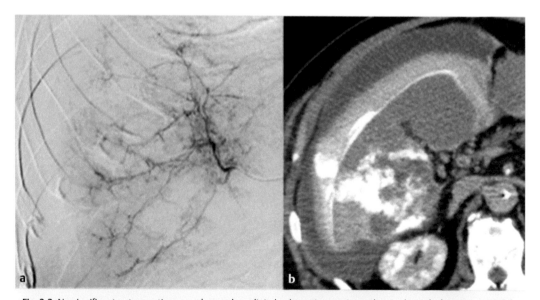

Fig. 3.3 No significant extravasation was observed on digital subtraction angiography via the right hepatic artery (a); however, significant extravasation was seen on CT during hepatic arteriography via the posterior segmental artery (b).

significant finding of extravasation on DSA. However, his vital signs were not improved after the second angiography.

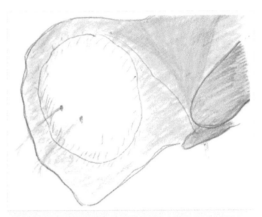

Fig. 3.4 Intraoperative view. Nonpulsatile bleeding indicated in red form biopsy sites was visible on the liver surface (*hand drawing*).

Possible Strategies for Complication Management

- Third angiography and embolization of the right hepatic artery.
- Percutaneous radiofrequency ablation around the biopsy site.
- Surgical hemostasis under the laparotomy.

Final Complication Management

Surgical laparotomy was performed. Nonpulsatile bleeding from two biopsy sites was observed, and surgical hemostasis was carried out with electric scalpel (▶ Fig. 3.4).

Complication Analysis

Bleeding complications after liver biopsy might be somewhat challenging to handle. A multidisciplinary approach might be warranted in dedicated cases.

Strategies to Prevent and Take-Home Message

- Percutaneous biopsy of liver tumor should be done with guiding needle to reduce the number of punctured hole on liver surface.
- Keep in mind that the liver receives blood supply not only from hepatic artery and portal vein, but also from many communicating vessels such as the isolated artery and the capsular arterial plexus. Therefore, the hepatic arterial embolization is not always effective to stop the bleeding from the liver.
- If hepatic arterial embolization is not effective for bleeding from the liver, surgical repair should be considered without delay.

Further Reading

Yoshida K, Matsui O, Miyayama S, et al. Isolated arteries originating from the intrahepatic arteries: anatomy, function, and importance in intervention. J Vasc Interv Radiol. 2018; 29(4): 531–537.e1

3.1.2 Hemothorax during Electroporation for Hepatocellular Carcinoma Treatment

Patient History

A 72-year-old female suffering from diabetes mellitus and cirrhosis related to metabolic disease, previously treated with hysterectomy and oophorectomy for endometrial cancer, underwent CT for a 2 cm hepatic nodule detected during surveillance with ultrasound. A hepatocellular carcinoma nodule of 2 cm involving hepatic segment 8/5 was demonstrated (▶ Fig. 3.5).

Initial Treatment

Due to her clinical comorbidities (including bilateral carotid stenosis)—a significant portal hypertension—a percutaneous approach was considered as the treatment of choice. The lesion was clearly visible at a pre-procedural ultrasound (▶ Fig. 3.6a) so the patient underwent percutaneous ultrasound-guided irreversible electroporation (▶ Fig. 3.6b) under general anesthesia.

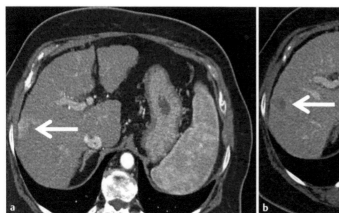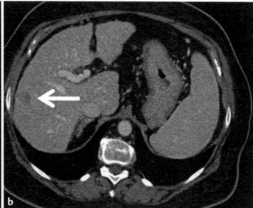

Fig. 3.5 (a) CT scans reveal a 2 cm subcapsular nodule occupying an area between the segments S8 and S5, slightly hyperdense in the arterial phase (*arrow*) and **(b)** hypodense in the portal venous phase (*arrow*).

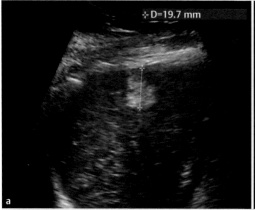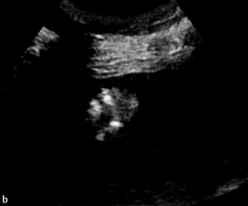

Fig. 3.6 The lesion is clearly visible at ultrasound **(a)**. Three electrodes of 15 cm length with 2 cm active tip are positioned, via intercostal space, to encompass the nodule **(b)**.

Problems Encountered during the Treatment

During the treatment time (about 5 minutes) irregular rhythm was observed, with bradyarrhythmia alternating with tachyarrhythmia. No specific treatment was given; blood pressure and O_2 saturation remained stable.

At the end of treatment, the patient reported severe pain, accentuated by breathing, not responding to ketorolac (45 mg) and tramadol (100 mg) administered intravenously. PO_2 was reduced (97 under O_2 administration).

Imaging Plan

Immediately after the procedure, the patient underwent CT, revealing right basal pleural effusion, with a density of more than 25 HU (▶ Fig. 3.7). After contrast administration, two small blushes of contrast were seen near the two ribs (VII and IX right rib) in the arterial acquisition, increased in the venous phase (▶ Fig. 3.8).

Resulting Complication

Hemothorax due to the puncture of an intercostal artery. No significant decrease in hemoglobin was observed.

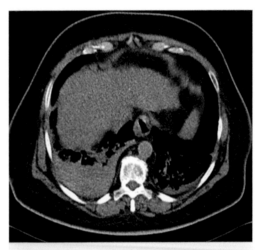

Fig. 3.7 Unenhanced CT scans reveal right basal pleural effusion, with a density greater than 25 HU.

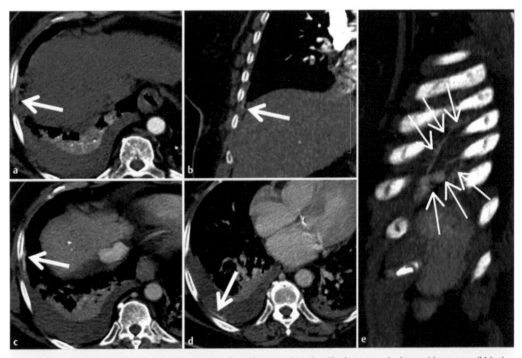

Fig. 3.8 *Thick arrows* point at the blood leakage at the right VII and IX ribs. The lesions, only detectable as a small blush in the arterial phase (**a–b**), increase in size in the venous phase (**c–d**). Multiplanar reconstruction (**e**) helps to confirm the diagnosis (*thin arrows*).

What Would You Do?

Notes:

_____

_____

_____

_____

_____

_____

_____

_____

Possible Strategies for Complication Management

- Conservative management (intensive care surveillance).
- Percutaneous drainage.
- Transcatheter embolization.
- Surgery.

Final Complication Management

Conservative management: patient was transferred to the intensive care unit the next day because she showed increased pain and severe dyspnea, decreased hemoglobin (–3 mg/dL), O_2 saturation (95 under O_2 administration), and increased size of hemothorax at chest X-ray (▶ Fig. 3.9).

The patient was then subjected to blood transfusion and percutaneous drainage of 600 cc of hemorrhagic fluid, with a clear improvement in her clinical picture. She was discharged 10 days later.

Complication Analysis

Sometimes it is rather difficult to determine the exact pathway during intercostal puncture, even

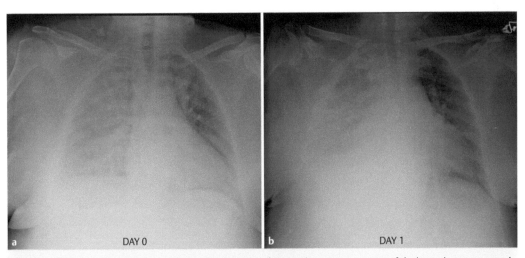

a   DAY 0
b   DAY 1

Fig. 3.9 Chest X-ray, performed the day after the procedure (**b**), reveals an increase in size of the hemothorax compared to the one taken right after the procedure (**a**).

when one is aware of the anatomy and the knowledge to pass the needle and any other device on the upper margin of the rib rather than on the lower margin of the rib above. The exact pathway is more difficult to predict in obese patients with an increased body mass index, as the case with the current patient.

Strategies to Prevent and Take-Home Message

- Intercostal artery bleeding represents a rather common complication after percutaneous thoracic procedures, with major bleeding only in a few patients.

- Management of intercostal artery bleeding events includes transcatheter embolization, with conservative management planned only in stable patients with minor lesions.
- Be sure that the needle is inserted over the top of the rib (superior margin) to avoid the intercostal nerves and blood vessels that run on the underside of the rib.

Further Reading

Pieper M, Schmitz J, McBane R, et al. Bleeding complications following image-guided percutaneous biopsies in patients taking clopidogrel: a retrospective review. J Vasc Interv Radiol. 2017; 28(1):88–93

Broderick SR. Hemothorax: etiology, diagnosis, and management. Thorac Surg Clin. 2013; 23(1):89–96, vi–vii

3.1.3 Cervical Hematoma after Thyroid Fine Needle Aspiration Biopsy

Patient History

A 52-year-old patient was diagnosed with a thyroid nodule during physical examination, which was confirmed on follow-up ultrasound (▶ Fig. 3.10, ▶ Fig. 3.11, ▶ Fig. 3.12).

Initial Treatment

To further evaluate the thyroid nodule, a fine needle aspiration biopsy was conducted under ultrasound guidance (22G). Three samples were obtained.

Problems Encountered during the Treatment

The patient developed neck swelling and dyspnea after procedure.

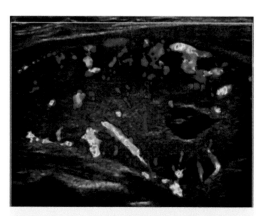

Fig. 3.10 Color Doppler ultrasound demonstrates a hypervascular nodule within the right thyroid lobe.

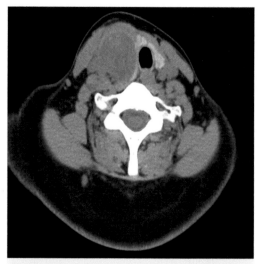

Fig. 3.11 CT scan of the neck shows an extensive cervical hematoma, likely within the right thyroid lobe resulting in left warded tracheal deviation.

Imaging Plan

A CT scan of the neck soft tissue was performed, which demonstrated right cervical hemorrhage associated with left-warded deviation of the trachea.

Resulting Complication

An extensive post-procedure right cervical hematoma, within the right thyroid lobe, was developed after the procedure.

What Would You Do?

Notes:

_____

_____

_____

_____

_____

_____

_____

_____

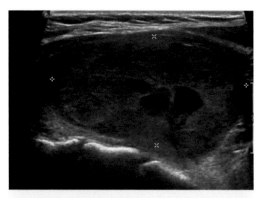

Fig. 3.12 B-mode ultrasound of the large nodule within the entire right thyroid lobe.

Complication Analysis

Insufficient compression over the punctuation site could result in post-biopsy hemorrhage and subsequent hematoma within the thyroid gland.

Strategies to Prevent and Take-Home Message

- Medication list should be checked before any intervention and adjusted appropriately.
- International normalized ratio and platelet levels should be determined before any intervention. Patients with increased risk of bleeding should be addressed accordingly with vitamin K substitution, cryoprecipitate, or fresh frozen plasma before biopsy or while encountering bleeding.
- Fine needle aspiration should never be conducted without ultrasound surveillance.
- Compression over the punctuation site should be performed to minimize the risk of post-procedural hemorrhage.

Possible Strategies for Complication Management

- Breathing support.
- Surgical exploration of the neck and drainage of the hematoma.

Final Complication Management

The surgical exploration of the neck revealed a large hematoma in the neck soft tissue without the evidence of active hemorrhage.

Further Reading

Ha EJ, Baek JH, Lee JH, et al. Complications following US-guided core-needle biopsy for thyroid lesions: a retrospective study of 6,169 consecutive patients with 6,687 thyroid nodules. Eur Radiol. 2017; 27(3):1186–1194

Akbaba G, Omar M, Polat M, et al. Cutaneous sinus formation is a rare complication of thyroid fine needle aspiration biopsy. Case Rep Endocrinol. 2014; 2014:923438

Lee YJ, Kim DW, Jung SJ. Comparison of sample adequacy, pain-scale ratings, and complications associated with ultrasound-guided fine-needle aspiration of thyroid nodules between two radiologists with different levels of experience. Endocrine. 2013; 44(3):696–701

Noordzij JP, Goto MM. Airway compromise caused by hematoma after thyroid fine-needle aspiration. Am J Otolaryngol. 2005; 26 (6):398–399

3.1.4 Hepatic Intraparenchymal Hemorrhage after CT-Guided Liver Biopsy

Patient History

A 55-year-old male with suspected hepatitis was scheduled for liver biopsy. No further comorbidities were present.

Initial Treatment and Imaging Plan

CT-guided percutaneous liver biopsy (16G).

Problems Encountered during the Treatment

The patient tolerated the procedure well, without any complication. The patient was discharged home.

Resulting Complication

The patient arrived to emergency room 6 hours after discharge, complaining of abdominal pain. On the physical examination, the patient was found to have tachycardia and hypotension. Contrast-enhanced CT scan of the abdomen revealed a hepatic intraparenchymal hemorrhage (▶ Fig. 3.13, ▶ Fig. 3.14, ▶ Fig. 3.15, ▶ Fig. 3.16).

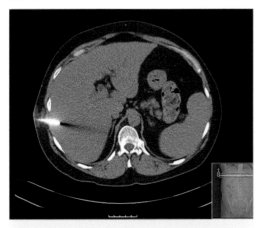

Fig. 3.13 CT-guided percutaneous liver biopsy shows the need biopsy aiming to the right hepatic lobe.

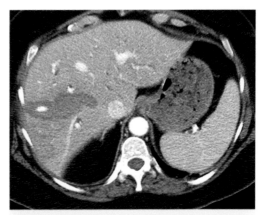

Fig. 3.14 Follow-up contrast-enhanced CT scan of abdomen demonstrates a small bilobulated hypodensity with small focus of hyperdensity in the right hepatic lobe, representing the hepatic intraparenchymal hematoma.

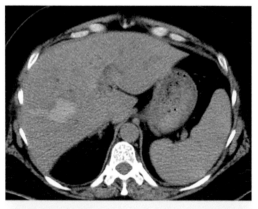

Fig. 3.15 Noncontrast CT scan of abdomen represents a hyperdense area in the right hepatic lobe, reflecting the hepatic intraparenchymal hematoma.

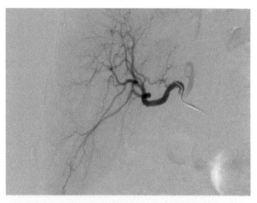

Fig. 3.16 Angiography of the right hepatic artery demonstrates no active contrast extravasation.

What Would You Do?

Notes:

_____

_____

_____

_____

_____

_____

_____

_____

Possible Strategies for Complication Management

- Conservative treatment.
- Local injection of Gelfoam immediately after biopsy.
- Embolization of the feeding vessel by using a microcatheter, selective injection of Gelfoam, glue, large particles, or coil.
- Surgical ligation (if an endovascular approach fails).

Final Complication Management

Angiography of hepatic vessels revealed no active hemorrhage. The patient was treated conservatively without embolization.

Complication Analysis

A small branch of the right hepatic artery was likely injured during the procedure, resulting in hemorrhage and hematoma. However, the hematoma remained undetected on the post-biopsy scan. The patient presented with symptomatic hemodynamic instability later.

Strategies to Prevent and Take-Home Message

- Medications should be checked before any intervention and adjusted appropriately.
- International normalized ratio and platelet levels should be determined before the intervention. Patients who are at increased risk of bleeding may benefit from vitamin K substitution, fresh frozen plasma, and cryoprecipitate before biopsy.
- Post-biopsy scan of the entire liver should be obtained.
- Patient's vital signs should be monitored at least for 2 to 4 hours post-biopsy.

Further Reading

Sag AA, Brody LA, Maybody M, et al. Acute and delayed bleeding requiring embolization after image-guided liver biopsy in patients with cancer. Clin Imaging. 2016; 40(3):535–540

Bishehsari F, Ting PS, Green RM. Recurrent gastrointestinal bleeding and hepatic infarction after liver biopsy. World J Gastroenterol. 2014; 20(7):1878–1881

Bannas P, Habermann CR, Yamamura J, Bley TA. Severe haemorrhage after liver biopsy of malignant B-cell lymphoma mimicking hepatic infection. RoFo Fortschr Geb Rontgenstr Nuklearmed. 2013; 185 (2):164–166

3.1.5 Hemodynamic Instability, Presumed to be Related to Worsening Retroperitoneal Hemorrhage during and after Cryoablation for Renal Tumor Treatment

Patient History

A 67-year-old female with a growing 4.2 cm left upper pole renal mass was scheduled for percutaneous cryoablation of her tumor because of her significant medical comorbidities. Given the size of the tumor, a preablative embolization to minimize the risk of bleeding was scheduled.

Initial Treatment and Imaging Plan

Initial left renal angiography via left radial arterial access demonstrated no clear vascular supply to the targeted lesion. A small round blush was seen related to an adrenal branch from the left renal capsular artery, which was thought to represent the targeted tumor. Attempts were made to embolize this lesion; however, the catheter kept spontaneously sliding out of the selected branch, and after multiple attempts, the catheter was only able to be transiently seated in the targeted vessel. About 1/20 of one vial of 100 to 300 µm Embospheres was injected before the catheter popped out again. No further embolization attempts were performed, and the decision was made to proceed with CT-guided cryoablation. The patient was then intubated electively due to poor baseline respiratory status. The patient was placed in the prone position in the CT scanner, and then four IceForce probes

(Galil Medical Inc., Arden Hills, MN, USA) were inserted through the left flank into the targeted tumor. Cryoablation proceeded with two 10-minute freeze cycles and an intervening 8-minute thaw cycle. The probes were then removed.

Problems Encountered during the Treatment

During the procedure, a moderate-sized retroperitoneal hematoma developed. Its size remained stable at the end of the procedure and the patient was hemodynamically stable throughout. At the end of the procedure, the patient was sent to the post-anesthesia recovery unit, where she was extubated. She then exhibited profound hypotension requiring vasopressor support. Due to her instability, no follow-up CT scan could be performed. Instead she was reintubated, and brought back to interventional radiology for angiography and embolization of a presumed worsening retroperitoneal hemorrhage.

Resulting Complication

Hypotension and hemodynamic instability, presumed to be related to worsening retroperitoneal hemorrhage (▶ Fig. 3.17, ▶ Fig. 3.18, ▶ Fig. 3.19, ▶ Fig. 3.20).

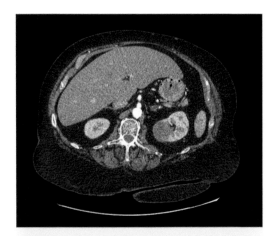

Fig. 3.17 Contrast-enhanced CT scan of the abdomen demonstrates a round hypodense mass in the right kidney upper pole before the treatment.

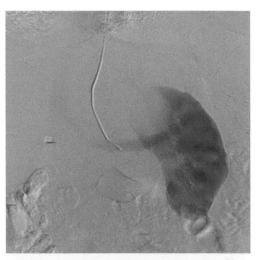

Fig. 3.18 The follow-up angiography reveals the right renal upper pole mass is hypovascular.

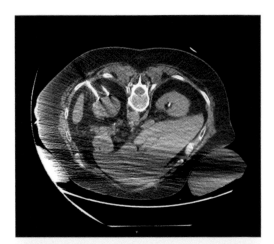

Fig. 3.19 Nonenhanced CT scan of abdomen shows two parallel cryoablation probes located within the right renal upper pole mass. The patient is in the prone position.

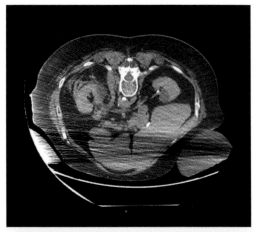

Fig. 3.20 The post-ablation CT scan of the abdomen shows the final extent of the postablation hematoma. The patient is in the prone position.

What Would You Do?

Notes:

_____

_____

_____

_____

_____

_____

_____

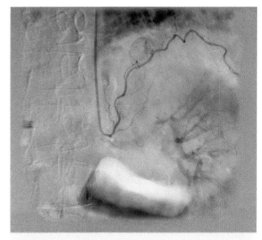

Fig. 3.21 Angiography demonstrates a capsular artery, which was thought to represent the targeted tumor.

Possible Strategies for Complication Management

- Catheterization of the feeding vessel, for example, by using a microcatheter, followed by selective coil embolization.
- Alternative agents for embolization: glue, large particles, Gelfoam.
- Surgery (if an endovascular approach fails).

Final Complication Management

Angiography including the aorta, left renal artery, left inferior phrenic artery, upper left lumbar arteries, lower left intercostal arteries, and capsular branch of the left renal artery was performed, showing no evidence of active extravasation. Empiric embolization to stasis of the capsular branch of the left renal artery using 100 to 300 μm Embospheres (Merit Medical, Jordan, UT, USA) was performed. Postembolization CT in retrospect showed no evidence of expansion of the hematoma compared to the scan ablation images, refuting the initial assumption that hypotension had

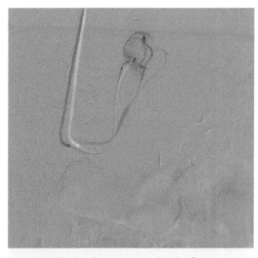

Fig. 3.22 The beads were injected under fluoroscopic guidance.

resulted from worsening hemorrhage. The next day, the patient was extubated and discharged home without event.

Complication Analysis

The initial angiography demonstrated a small subbranch of the capsular branch supplying a small rounded tumor. At the time, it was thought that this tumor was a component of the patient's large renal cell carcinoma (▶ Fig. 3.21, ▶ Fig. 3.22).

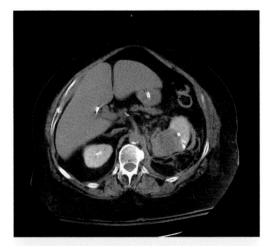

Fig. 3.23 Nonenhanced CT scan of abdomen demonstrates the postablation hematoma and perinephric inflammatory changes.

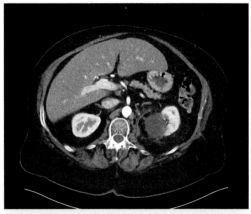

Fig. 3.24 One-month follow-up contrast-enhanced CT scan of the upper abdomen demonstrates the ablation cavity within the right renal upper pole with interval significant improvement of the perinephric inflammatory stranding.

However, this lesion in retrospect represented the patient's known left adrenal nodule, embolization of which may have resulted in hypoadrenergic state and caused hypotension. Alternatively, her episode may have been related to anesthesia.

Strategies to Prevent and Take-Home Message

- Consider the reasonability of embolization of hypovascular tumors (▶ Fig. 3.23, ▶ Fig. 3.24).

Further Reading

Schmit GD, Schenck LA, Thompson RH, et al. Predicting renal cryoablation complications: new risk score based on tumor size and location and patient history. Radiology. 2014; 272(3):903–910

Chen JX, Guzzo TJ, Malkowicz SB, et al. Complication and readmission rates following same-day discharge after percutaneous renal tumor ablation. J Vasc Interv Radiol. 2016; 27(1):80–86

Atwell TD, Carter RE, Schmit GD, et al. Complications following 573 percutaneous renal radiofrequency and cryoablation procedures. J Vasc Interv Radiol. 2012; 23(1):48–54

3.1.6 Mediastinal Hemorrhage and Hemothorax after Anterior Mediastinal Puncture

Patient History

A 48-year-old male was scheduled for biopsy of an anterior mediastinal mass. The patient had no further comorbidities.

Initial Treatment and Imaging Plan

CT-guided percutaneous biopsy was performed using an 18-gauge coaxial biopsy system through parasternal approach.

Problems Encountered during the Treatment

The patient developed tachycardia and hypotension during the treatment.

Resulting Complication

CT scan of the chest demonstrated a mediastinal hemorrhage and hemothorax (▶ Fig. 3.25, ▶ Fig. 3.26, ▶ Fig. 3.27, ▶ Fig. 3.28).

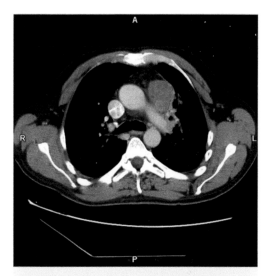

Fig. 3.25 Contrast-enhanced CT scan of the chest shows the anterior mediastinal mass before the intervention.

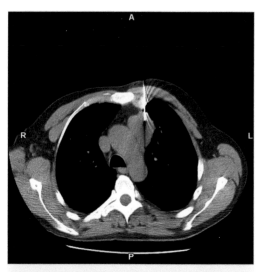

Fig. 3.26 CT-guided percutaneous biopsy of the anterior mediastinal mass demonstrates the coaxial biopsy system terminating in the mass through parasternal approach.

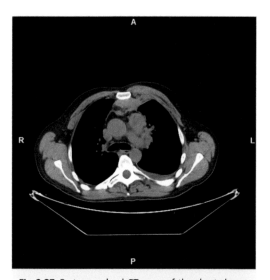

Fig. 3.27 Post-procedural CT scans of the chest shows mediastinal hematoma and small left hemithorax.

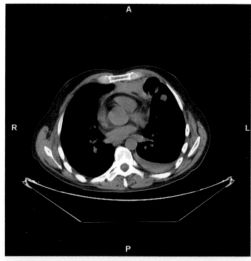

Fig. 3.28 Post-procedural CT scans of chest shows the final extent of the hematoma and left hemothorax.

What Would You Do?

Notes:

_____

_____

_____

_____

_____

_____

_____

Complication Analysis

The biopsy needle injured the internal mammary artery, leading to the hemorrhage. Alternatively, the bleeding might originate from the mass itself or from the pleura.

Strategies to Prevent and Take-Home Message

- Contrast-enhanced CT or MRI should be obtained before the biopsy. Careful anatomical evaluation is necessary to identify abutting vascular lesions.
- For vascularized lesions, needles with small diameter should be utilized to minimize the risk of vascular injury and hemorrhage.
- The internal mammary vessels can be preserved by aiming medial to the vessels and advancing needle adjacent to the sternum or lateral to the vessels.
- Injection of contrast during procedure may help to better determine the anatomical structures and differentiate lymph nodes and vasculature.
- Patients should be observed for 1 to 3 hours after procedure.

Possible Strategies for Complication Management

- Conservative treatment.
- Selective embolization of the supplying vessel by Gelfoam, glue, large particles, or coil using a microcatheter.
- Surgical ligation (if the endovascular approach fails).

Final Complication Management

The patient was treated conservatively.

Further Reading

Barker JM, Sahn SA. Opacified hemithorax with ipsilateral mediastinal shift after transthoracic needle biopsy. Chest. 2003; 124(6):2391–2392

Giron J, Fajadet P, Senac JP, Durand G, Benezet O, Didier A. [Diagnostic percutaneous thoracic punctures. Assessment through a critical study of a compilation of 2406 cases]. Rev Mal Respir. 1996; 13(6):583–590

Berquist TH, Bailey PB, Cortese DA, Miller WE. Transthoracic needle biopsy: accuracy and complications in relation to location and type of lesion. Mayo Clin Proc. 1980; 55(8):475–481

3.1.7 Hemoptysis after Percutaneous Lung Biopsy

Patient History

A 75-year-old immunocompromised patient presented with a clinical history of chronic dyspnea. Conventional radiography and follow-up contrast-enhanced CT of the chest showed a left paramediastinal mass, raising a concern for tuberculosis.

Initial Treatment

A CT-guided percutaneous lung biopsy using an 18-gauge coaxial biopsy system was performed to obtain a tissue sample (▶ Fig. 3.29).

Problems Encountered during the Treatment

Subsequent to the biopsy, the patient developed hemoptysis.

Imaging Plan

A CT angiography of the chest was immediately performed demonstrating a left lower lobe segmental pulmonary artery pseudoaneurysm.

Resulting Complication

A pulmonary artery injury could happen as a complication of biopsy. In this case, a pseudoaneurysm of the left lower lobe segmental pulmonary artery occurred during biopsy (▶ Fig. 3.30, ▶ Fig. 3.31, ▶ Fig. 3.32).

What Would You Do?
Notes:

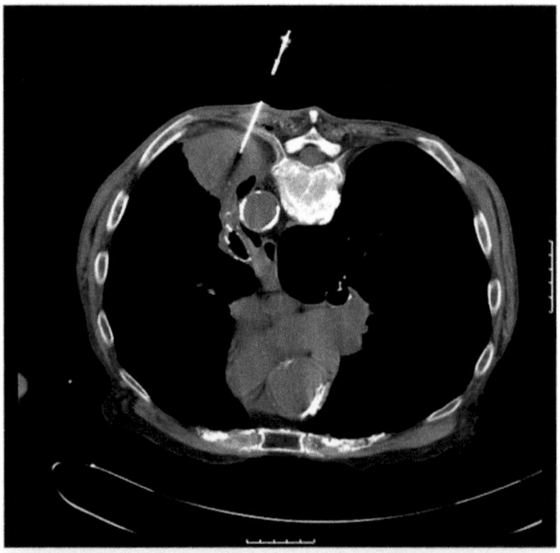

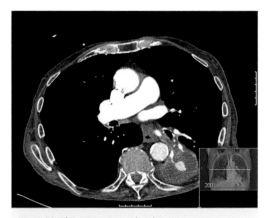

Fig. 3.29 CT-guided percutaneous lung biopsy was performed by a coaxial biopsy system with the distal tip of the needle within the left paravertebral mass.

Fig. 3.30 The CT angiography shows a pseudoaneurysm in the left lower lobe segmental pulmonary artery.

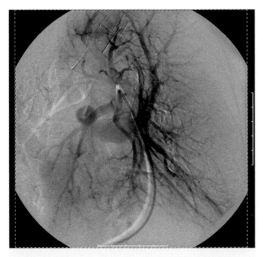

Fig. 3.31 Angiography shows the sacular dilatation of the left lower lobe segmental pulmonary artery.

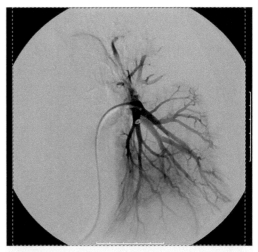

Fig. 3.32 Angiography of the left common basal artery demonstrates complete coil embolization of the left lower lobe segmental pseudoaneurysm.

Possible Strategies for Complication Management

- Embolization of the pseudoaneurysm using Gelfoam, glue, or coil.

Final Complication Management

Initial selective angiography was performed to determine the anatomical location of the pseudoaneurysm. Embolization of the pseudoaneurysm was then performed by packing microcoils within the pseudoaneurysm sac. Finally, complete occlusion of the pseudoaneurysm sac was yielded.

Complication Analysis

A pulmonary artery was injured during the percutaneous lung biopsy, resulting in development of pseudoaneurysm.

Strategies to Prevent and Take-Home Message

- Post biopsy cross-sectional images should be obtained immediately after removing the biopsy needle.
- The patient's vital signs should be monitored at least for 2 hours.

Further Reading

Hwang EJ, Park CM, Yoon SH, Lim HJ, Goo JM. Risk factors for haemoptysis after percutaneous transthoracic needle biopsies in 4,172 cases: Focusing on the effects of enlarged main pulmonary artery diameter. Eur Radiol. 2018; 28(4):1410–1419

Heerink WJ, de Bock GH, de Jonge GJ, Groen HJ, Vliegenthart R, Oudkerk M. Complication rates of CT-guided transthoracic lung biopsy: meta-analysis. Eur Radiol. 2017; 27(1):138–148

Tai R, Dunne RM, Trotman-Dickenson B, et al. Frequency and severity of pulmonary hemorrhage in patients undergoing percutaneous CT-guided transthoracic lung biopsy: single-institution experience of 1175 cases. Radiology. 2016; 279 (1):287–296

3.1.8 Delayed Bleeding after Biliary Drainage

Patient History

A 70-year-old female with history of unresectable pancreatic tumor was admitted to the emergency room with jaundice, fever, and dull abdominal pain. CT scan showed a 2 cm lesion (▶ Fig. 3.33a) of the uncinated process of the pancreas, with encasement of superior mesenteric artery (▶ Fig. 3.33b), undissociable from the third portion of the duodenum (▶ Fig. 3.33c), with compression of the Vater papilla and subsequent dilation of the intra- and extrahepatic biliary tree (▶ Fig. 3.33b–d). Laboratory examination revealed high value of bilirubin (12 mg/dL), liver enzymes (especially GGT: 320 U/L, normal values: 12–48 U/L), and CA19.9 (800 U/mL, normal values < 35 U/mL).

Initial Treatment

To reduce cholestasis, an 8 French internal–external drainage (▶ Fig. 3.34) was placed through ultrasound puncture of the segment 3 biliary duct, with its apex in the duodenum, passing papillary stenosis.

Problems Encountered during the Treatment

No immediate complication was demonstrated; in particular amylase/lipase levels remained in the normal range. Bilirubin values progressively decreases and the patient was discharged 4 days later (bilirubin 3 mg/dL).

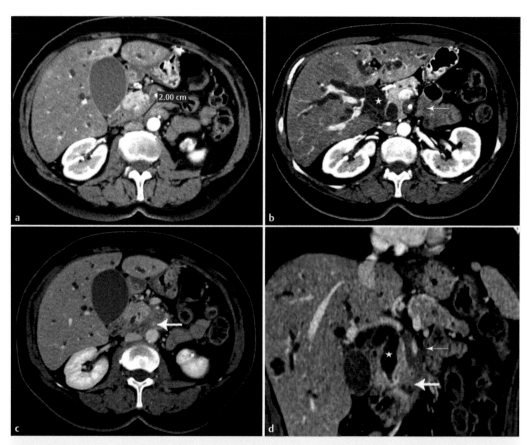

Fig. 3.33 CT reveals a 2 cm lesion (**a**) of the uncinate process of the pancreas, with encasement of 3 cm of the proximal tract of SMA (**b**, *thin arrow*), undissociable from the third portion of the duodenum (**c**, *thick arrow*), with dilation of the intra and extra-hepatic biliary tree (**b, d**, *star*).

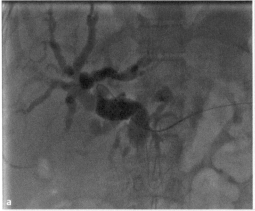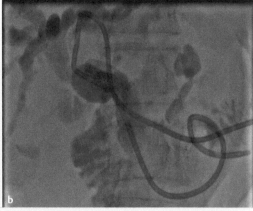

Fig. 3.34 Placement of 8 French internal–external biliary drainage: overcoming of the papillary stenosis with a stiff guidewire **(a)** and evaluation of the correct placement of the drainage after the percutaneous procedure **(b)**.

Imaging Plan

Ultrasound in order to gain any information about the progress of drainage; in case of limited information due to artifacts like bowel air, a contrast-enhanced CT will be scheduled.

Resulting Complication

Two weeks after the procedure, due to liver enzyme increase, the internal–external drainage was replaced first with a 10 French and then with a 12 French.

One month after the procedure the patient was admitted to the emergency room, with gross haemobilia. Laboratory examination showed low hemoglobin level (8 g/dL, normal values: 3.5–17.5 g/dL).

Possible Strategies for Complication Management

- Conservative treatment (surveillance, with hemoglobin evaluation every 6 hours).
- CT evaluation.
- Review and eventual replacement of the biliary drainage.
- Surgery.

What Would You Do?

Notes:

_____

_____

_____

_____

_____

_____

_____

_____

_____

Final Complication Management

Evaluation of the biliary drainage: during the drainage removal a jet blood leak was demonstrated and contrast injection through the sheath showed an arterial leakage (▶ Fig. 3.35a).

Catheterization of celiac trunk was performed with a 5 French reverse curve catheter, with a 3 French microcatheter a leak from the segment 4 hepatic artery (▶ Fig. 3.35b), and a communication between the biliary tree and the segmental hepatic artery were revealed. The small leakage was treated with absorbable gel foam and detachable coil embolization (▶ Fig. 3.35c).

After the procedure a 14 French internal–external biliary drainage (▶ Fig. 3.35d) was placed.

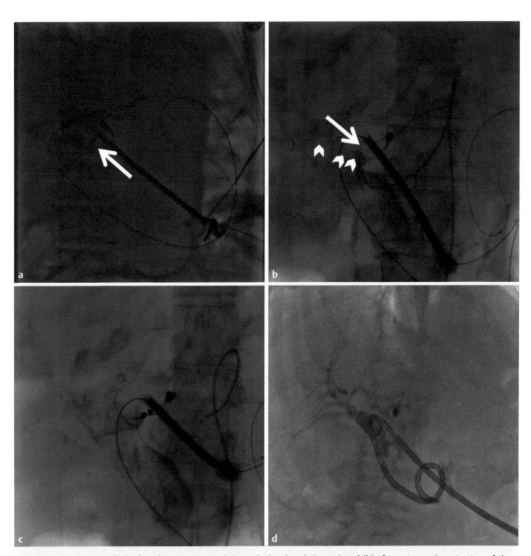

Fig. 3.35 (a) Contrast leak after drainage removal through the sheath (*arrow*) and **(b)** after microcatheterization of the segment 4 hepatic artery (*arrow*) confirms the small arterial leakage, with biliary tree evidence (*arrowheads*). **(c)** The image shows absence of blood leak after coil embolization; after the procedure a 4 French internal–external biliary drainage **(d)** was placed.

Complication Analysis

Iatrogenic injuries secondary to percutaneous biliary drain placement are rare, usually manifesting 1 to 7 days after the procedure; vascular bleeding, instead, is a late finding and the only symptom may be persistent hemobilia.

Hemobilia may be due to arterial or venous bleeding. In each case, the interventional radiologist may embolize (gel foam and coils) the offending vessel, with other alternatives being balloon tamponade or stent placement. Aggressive arterial embolization may lead to vascular compromise, especially in the setting of portal vein occlusion, so the interventional radiologist should be aware of this further complication.

Strategies to Prevent and Take-Home Message

A careful follow-up of the patient is of utmost importance since iatrogenic injuries secondary to percutaneous biliary drain placement are rare and usually occur 1 to 7 days after the procedure.

Further Reading

Ernst O, Sergent G, Mizrahi D, Delemazure O, L'Herminé C. Biliary leaks: treatment by means of percutaneous transhepatic biliary drainage. Radiology. 1999; 211(2):345–348

Born P, Rösch T, Sandschin W, Weiss W. Arterial bleeding as an unusual late complication of percutaneous transhepatic biliary drainage. Endoscopy. 2003; 35(11):978–979

Lynskey GE, Banovac F, Chang T. Vascular complications associated with percutaneous biliary drainage: a report of three cases. Semin Intervent Radiol. 2007; 24(3):316–319

3.1.9 Bleeding during Diagnostic CT-Guided Liver Puncture

Patient History

A 74-year-old male patient with a 10 cm lesion of the right liver lobe, involving segments 5 and 6 was scheduled for CT-guided diagnostic puncture in order to obtain the exact diagnosis. Due to medical history and laboratory changes, a hepatocellular carcinoma was suspected. Diagnostic-enhanced CT scan has depicted a hypodense lesion with some enhancing vessel-like appearing areas inside (▶ Fig. 3.36). Native T1 MRI showed a larger appearance of the lesion reaching to the liver capsule. The high intense signal of the main lesion was interpreted as products of blood (▶ Fig. 3.37).

Initial Treatment

So far no treatment was done. The diagnostic procedure was planned for further diagnostic reasons in order to offer the patient an individualized treatment concept.

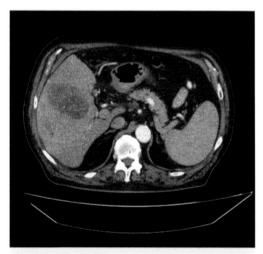

Fig. 3.36 Contrast-enhanced axial CT-scan of the right liver lobe showing a 9 cm hypodense lesion surrounded by a hyperdense zone involving most parts of segment 6. The lesion reaches to the liver capsule without penetrating it.

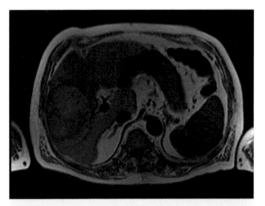

Fig. 3.37 Native axial T1 MRI presenting the lesion of the right liver lobe, appearing much larger as in the previous CT. No signs of infiltration or penetration of surrounding structures such as vessels and liver capsule are visible.

Diagnostic puncture was done under local anesthesia with 10 mL Prilocaine hydrochloride 1%. The body was elevated for 45 degrees in order to start percutaneous access in the posterior axillary line. After skin incision, 16G 6 cm trocar (Quick-Core Biopsy Needle Set, Cook, Bloomington, IN, USA) was inserted and after checking the adequate position, an 18G 9 cm biopsy needle was inserted and 5 probes were successfully taken.

Problems Encountered during the Treatment

After the last probe, some pulsatile bleeding through the trocar needle appeared.

Imaging Plan

No initial imaging was planned to beat the bleeding complication.

Resulting Complication

Bleeding during diagnostic liver puncture.

What Would You Do?

Notes:

_____

_____

_____

_____

_____

_____

_____

_____

Possible Strategies for Complication Management

- Retrograde puncture of the femoral groin. Placement of a 4 French sheath into the ipsilateral common femoral artery. Catheterization of the coeliac trunk with 4 French Cobra catheter and performing diagnostic angiography in order to visualize a potential bleeding source, that is, coming from right hepatic artery branches. If this would be the case, an embolization procedure (coils, glue, particles) via a coaxially placed microcatheter could be performed.
- Embolization via the trocar using gel foam until the bleeding stops.
- Surgical, laparoscopic evaluation, and potential treatment of the source of the bleeding.

Final Complication Management

Embolization via the trocar using gel foam until the bleeding stops.

Complication Analysis

During puncture and biopsy vessel damage occurred, either a portal vein branch or a hepatic artery branch, resulting in permanent bleeding trough the inserted trocar. Due to the fact that nearly no covering regular liver tissue between malignant lesion and liver capsule existed, the risk of intraperitoneal bleeding is slightly higher than with a zone of nondiseased tissue in between.

Strategies to Prevent and Take-Home Message

- Handle instruments with care. Try to find a way to reach the lesion through a surrounding zone of nondiseased liver tissue. This will prevent, in case of vessel injury, a significant bleeding through the puncture channel, since the nondiseased tissue will close this channel rather fast in case of minor, low pressure bleeding.
- In case of bleeding through the puncture needle, keep the needle stable in place and close the puncture channel mechanically. Before discharge, the puncture sites should be evaluated by ultrasound or native CT to check for any bleeding complications (hematoma, fluid intraperitoneal).
- The most critical aspect of management of complications such as bleeding, pneumothorax, and visceral perforation is to recognize that one these complications has occurred during liver biopsy.

Further Reading

van Beek D, Funaki B. Hemorrhage as a complication of percutaneous liver biopsy. Semin Intervent Radiol. 2013; 30(4):413–416

Sandrasegaran K, Thayalan N, Thavanesan R, et al. Risk factors for bleeding after liver biopsy. Abdom Radiol (NY). 2016; 41(4): 643–649

Kennedy SA, Milovanovic L, Midia M. Major bleeding after percutaneous image-guided biopsies: frequency, predictors, and periprocedural management. Semin Intervent Radiol. 2015; 32(1): 26–33

3.1.10 Bleeding after Radiofrequency Ablation for Hepatocellular Carcinoma Treatment

Patient History

An 80-year-old female patient was planned for percutaneous thermal ablation of subcapsular hepatocellular carcinoma in the second segment (▶ Fig. 3.38). She had a Child's class B without other comorbidities. Before the procedure, laboratory tests were evaluated, especially blood coagulation function, presenting normal values.

Initial Treatment

The patient was scheduled for radiofrequency ablation (RFA). RFA was performed using real-time ultrasound guidance under conscious sedation. Every effort was made in order to minimize the number of transgression of the liver capsule and to traverse sufficient normal liver parenchyma. Cauterization of the needle tract was also performed.

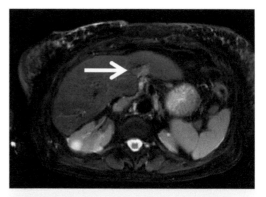

Fig. 3.38 MRI T2 fat saturated sequence shows a hyperintense nodular lesion in the second hepatic segment (*arrow*).

Problems Encountered during the Treatment

No complications were reported during the procedure, total necrosis of the tumor was achieved.

Imaging Plan

Contrast-enhanced CT performed as control check after 3 hours showed an active and massive abdominal bleeding (▶ Fig. 3.39) from an injured vessel posterior to the left liver lobe, suggesting rupture of the lesion.

What Would You Do?

Notes:

_____

_____

_____

_____

_____

_____

_____

_____

Possible Strategies for Complication Management

- Blood transfusion.
- Transarterial embolization.
- Surgery.

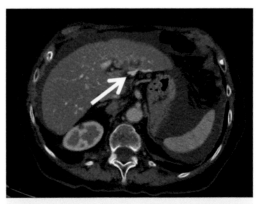

Fig. 3.39 Contrast-enhanced CT shows a massive intraperitoneal contrast blush posterior to the site of ablation (*arrow*). Massive intraperitoneal hypodense masses interpreted as the result of bleeding is also detected.

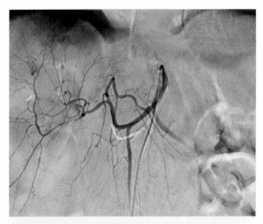

Fig. 3.40 Selective digital subtraction angiography of the hepatic vasculature, not showing any direct signs of bleeding.

Final Complication Management

Emergency transfemoral hepatic arterial embolization via transfemoral approach was performed as diagnostic (▶ Fig. 3.40) and therapeutic procedure. Immediately after the detection of the bleeding point (▶ Fig. 3.41), transarterial embolization was performed with microcoils (▶ Fig. 3.42). The bleeding was stopped, as also suggested by the improvement of the clinical and laboratory data.

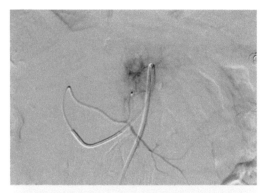

Fig. 3.41 Selective catheterization of the vessel feeding the site of ablation, showing direct sign of bleeding.

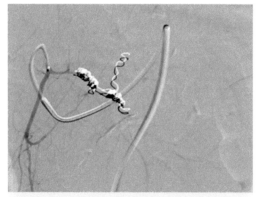

Fig. 3.42 Postembolization angiogram shows the placement of several coils at the site of active bleeding.

Complication Analysis

Hemorrhage is one of the most common major complications occurring during RFA. Several factors are related to bleeding. The most important risk factor in our case was the location of the lesion: it was subcapsular and adjacent to a major blood vessel injured due to direct mechanical trauma by electrode needle. Physician performing RFA have to pay attention to the localization of the lesion and they must be cognizant of the diagnosis and treatment of a possible bleeding.

Strategies to Prevent and Take-Home Message

- Screening for coagulopathy should be performed before RFA.
- It is important to be careful if the lesion is subcapsular, minimizing the number of transgressions of the liver capsule.

- An accurate monitoring of hemodynamic parameters during procedure is mandatory.
- Contrast-enhanced CT is the choice for the detection end evaluation of post-procedural bleeding, even if in some centers contrast-enhanced ultrasound is used for immediate post-procedural control.

Further Reading

Rhim H, Yoon KH, Lee JM, et al. Major complications after radiofrequency thermal ablation of hepatic tumors: spectrum of imaging findings. Radiographics. 2003; 23(1):123–134, discussion 134–136

Rhim H. Complications of radiofrequency ablation in hepatocellular carcinoma. Abdom Imaging. 2005; 30(4):409–418

Park JG, Park SY, Tak WY, et al. Early complications after percutaneous radiofrequency ablation for hepatocellular carcinoma: an analysis of 1,843 ablations in 1,211 patients in a single centre: experience over 10 years. Clin Radiol. 2017; 72(8):692.e9–692.e15

3.1.11 Massive Pleural Hemorrhage after Lung Radiofrequency Ablation

Patient History

A 57-year-old man with history of lung metastases for colorectal cancer had video assisted thoracic surgery for wedge resection of a single lung metastasis in the right upper lobe 20 months ago. Patient had a CT-guided radiofrequency in the right lower lobe 8 months ago for a single 12 mm lung metastasis. On follow-up CT-imaging, a scar

(*white arrow*) as well as a new location of lung metastasis in the right lower lobe (*red arrow*; ▶ Fig. 3.43a) can be seen. Tumor board decision was again in favor for RFA.

Initial Treatment

Lung RFA is performed under general anesthesia in the prone position. After single puncture, parave-

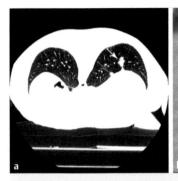
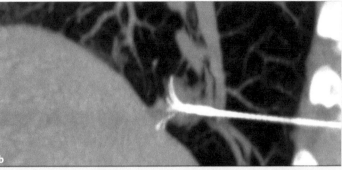

Fig. 3.43 **(a)** CT in the prone position demonstrates the radiofrequency ablation zone of the metastasis treated 8 months ago (*white arrow*) and the new metastasis (*red arrow*). **(b)** CT in the prone position demonstrates the LeVeen radiofrequency needle inserted in the targeted metastasis.

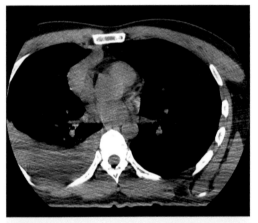

Fig. 3.44 CT in the supine position demonstrates large right pleural effusion.

rtebral placement of a LeVeen radiofrequency electrode was done successfully (Boston Scientific, Nattick, MA, USA) under CT guidance (▶ Fig. 3.43b).

Problems Encountered during the Treatment

After completion of RFA treatment, patient is placed in the supine position and a pleural effusion is seen; after 10 minutes of observation, a second CT scan is obtained while the blood pressure drops and the heart rate accelerates (▶ Fig. 3.44).

Resulting Complication

Massive pleural hemorrhage.

What Would You Do?

Notes:

_____

_____

_____

_____

_____

_____

_____

_____

Possible Strategies for Complication Management

- Watchful follow-up.
- Pleural drainage.
- Pulmonary angiogram.
- Bronchial angiogram.
- Intercostal angiogram.

Final Complication Management

Angiogram is performed in the same room (angio-CT room) with selective catheterization of right intercostal branches (*arrow*) running toward the vicinity at previous puncture site (▶ Fig. 3.45a). Extravasation of contrast to the pleura (*arrow*) is seen on the digital subtracted angiogram at a later phase (▶ Fig. 3.45b).

Coil embolization (*white arrows*) was performed in sandwich technique to stop arterial bleeding (*black arrow*; ▶ Fig. 3.45c).

Pleural drainage is then performed with a 26 French drainage catheter and aspiration of 700 cc of coagulated blood was also done (underlining the need for a very large size and lumen catheter). Patient recovered after 48 hours at the intensive care unit and was discharged at day 4 after treatment.

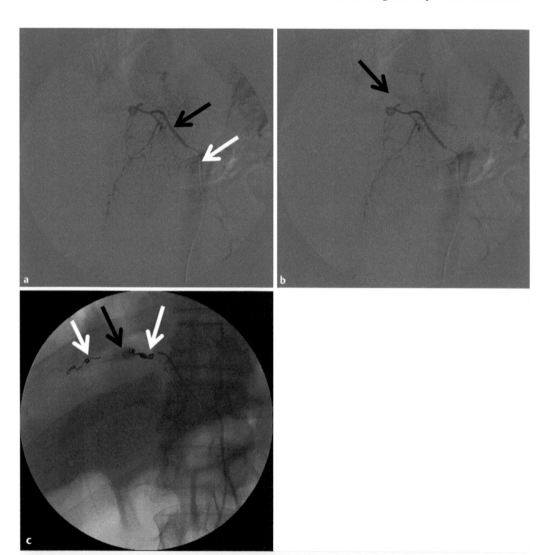

Fig. 3.45 (a) Digital subtraction angiography of the intercostal artery (*black arrow*) obtained with a 5 French catheter (*white arrow*). **(b)** Contrast extravasation (*black arrow*) shown at late phase scans. **(c)** X-ray obtained after coiling on the inflow (medial *white arrow*) and the outflow (lateral *white arrow*), while the microcatheter used for coil delivery is still in place in proximal part of the intercostal artery. The damage to the artery is still visible with extravasation of contrast to the segment of the artery in between the coils (*black arrow*).

Complication Analysis

Pleural hemorrhage due to intercostal artery damage during the puncture.

Strategies to Prevent and Take-Home Message

Accidental puncture of the intercostal artery might happen when performing diagnostic or therapeutic needle insertion into lung or pleura space. Any pleural effusion, which rapidly increases and diagnosed on control CT, must induce an angiogram for potential intervention like an embolization procedure. The risk of injuring the intercostal artery is higher when intercostal puncture is performed in the paravertebral region. Here the intercostal artery runs between the ribs without the protection from the bone of the lateral or anterior aspect of the ribs. During endovascular treatment of this complication, the curve of the guidewire is noted in the proximal part of the intercostal artery (*black arrow*), meaning it is running midway in between the ribs and the artery is prone for the risk of inadvertent puncture at this level, while on its more distal/peripheral part the subcostal artery pathway is below the ribs inferior margin (*white arrow*) with much lower risk of inadvertent puncture, especially if a puncture is performed immediately above the rib margin (▶ Fig. 3.46). When intercostal puncture is needed in the paravertebral area, a likely valid option to minimize the risk of harming the intercostal artery could be using a blunt needle when traversing the muscle.

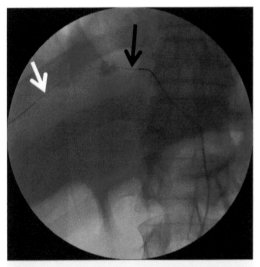

Fig. 3.46 The pathway of the intercostal artery is imaged by the guidewire placed in the intercostal artery. The middle/proximal segment is in the middle of the intercostal space (*black arrow*) where it is at risk for puncture because no bony landmark can help for puncture. The distal/peripheral segment of the intercostal artery is located under the ribs (*white arrow*) where it is relatively protected from puncture when the lower part of the intercostal space is targeted.

Further Reading

McAllister M, Lim K, Torrey R, Chenoweth J, Barker B, Baldwin DD. Intercostal vessels and nerves are at risk for injury during supracostal percutaneous nephrolithotomy. J Urol. 2011; 185 (1):329–334

Li BQ, Ye B, Chen FX, et al. Intercostal artery damage and massive hemothorax after thoracocentesis by central venous catheter: a case report. Chin J Traumatol. 2017; 20(5):305–307

Lai JH, Yan HC, Kao SJ, Lee SC, Shen CY. Intercostal arteriovenous fistula due to pleural biopsy. Thorax. 1990; 45(12):976–978

3.1.12 Delayed Bleeding after Microwave Ablation for a Recurrent Colorectal Liver Metastasis

Patient History

A 65-year-old male with metastatic colon carcinoma with prior liver resection, systemic and HAIP (hepatic arterial pump) chemotherapy, with new 20 × 23 × 30 mm recurrent metastasis at the surgical resection margin along the border of the left hemi-liver, detected on routine surveillance CT examination. On review of the case and multidisciplinary discussion, the patient was deemed a good candidate for thermal microwave (MW) ablation.

Initial Treatment

The patient underwent percutaneous MW ablation under general anesthesia as per standard clinical practice. The goal of the procedure was to treat the entire tumor with at least 1 cm circumferential minimal ablation margin. Since the tumor was (fluorodeoxyglucose) FDG-avid, the split-dose ^{18}F-FDG PET/CT technique was used for tumor

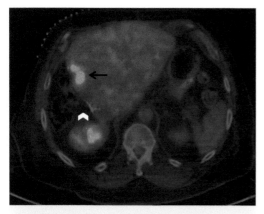

Fig. 3.47 Preablation ^{18}F-FDG PET/CT utilizing a split-dose protocol. The FDG-avid mass is again identified along the resection margin (*black arrow*). A loop of large bowel is seen directly adjacent to the liver (*white arrowhead*).

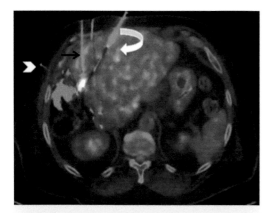

Fig. 3.48 Intra-procedural ^{18}F-FDG PET/CT imaging after placement of microwave ablation probes for overlapping ablation. The recurrent tumor is located at the surgical margin after the prior right hepatectomy. Three probes, two in plane are identified in the region of the tumor (*black arrow*). A temperature probe is placed at the desired margin for temperature monitoring and adjustment of ablation settings (*white curved arrow*). A needle was placed in the right upper quadrant adjacent to the liver for hydrodissection of the adjacent loops of the colon away from the ablation zone with a 1:10 solution of contrast and normal saline (*white arrowhead*).

localization, MW electrode placement, as well as confirmation of complete ablation and immediate assessment of technical success (▶ Fig. 3.47).

After careful imaging consideration, three overlapping ablations were performed utilizing three Neuwave PR 15 electrodes (Ethicon, Madison, Wisconsin, USA), with real-time prophylactic hydrodissection of the colon. The treatment protocol utilized for each ablation session was 65 W for a total of 6 minutes (two overlaps were performed with two electrodes, a third overlap ablation was performed with three electrodes), with temperature monitoring at the intended ablation margin (until reaching 70 °C; ▶ Fig. 3.48).

Pre- and postablation biopsies were performed within institution research protocol with specimens obtained from the ablation zone center, ablation margin, as well as from the electrodes. There was no evidence of viable tumor post-MW ablation.

Problems Encountered during the Treatment

None. Patient was successfully treated with MW ablation. Both immediate postablation ^{18}F-FDG PET/CT (▶ Fig. 3.49) and three-phase contrast-enhanced CT scans demonstrated complete ablation of the tumor, with ablation zone size of 60 × 45 × 50 mm.

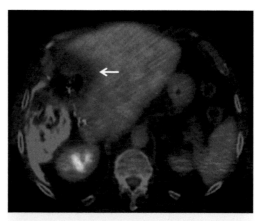

Fig. 3.49 Immediate postablation imaging to evaluate for technical success of microwave ablation. Split-dose ^{18}F-FDG PET/CT demonstrated no metabolic uptake in the previously FDG-avid tumor, with a central gas focus, related to tumor desiccation (*arrow*).

Imaging Plan

Patient was scheduled for multiphase abdominal CT scan within 4 to 6 weeks after ablation, in order to confirm technical success/complete ablation; this was to serve as the new baseline for future comparisons.

Resulting Complication

Three weeks after the procedure, the patient presented to interventional radiology clinic with vague right upper quadrant pain, radiating to the back. The patient had decreased hemoglobin concentration (8.6 g/dL, baseline level-12.3 g/dL), mild thrombocytopenia (136 K/mcl), and norman white blood cell count (4.6 K/mcl). A contrast-enhanced CT scan was obtained at that time, this demonstrated a 50 mm pseudoaneurysm within the ablation zone with active hemorrhage (▶ Fig. 3.50).

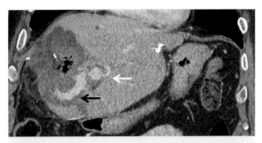

Fig. 3.50 Contrast-enhanced CT, reconstructed in the coronal plane, was obtained after patient complained of abdominal pain. *White arrow* indicates a pseudoaneurysm of the segment 4 hepatic artery branch. *Black arrow* identifies active arterial hemorrhage into the hypoattenuating ablation zone that is significantly bigger than on the day of the procedure.

What Would You Do?

Notes:

_____

_____

_____

_____

_____

_____

_____

_____

Possible Strategies for Complication Management

- Embolization of the pseudoaneurysm and feeding vessels.

- Covered stent placement isolating the pseudoaneurysm with possible embolization.
- Conservative "watch and wait" approach with close monitoring of the hemoglobin, hematocrit, and vital signs. However, it is not acceptable option in the case of active extravasation.
- Percutaneous or transcatheter thrombin injection within the pseudoaneurysm.

Final Complication Management

The patient was transferred to the hospital where he underwent a diagnostic angiogram and embolization.

Digital subtraction angiography (DSA) was performed in the celiac and proper hepatic arteries with a 5 French Simmons 2 catheter (Angiodynamic, Latham, NY, USA). Additionally, superselective DSA was performed within the segment 4 and segment 2/3 arteries using a renegade microcatheter (Boston Scientific, Marlborough, MA, USA). Multifocal extravasation of contrast medium was identified from the hepatic segment 4 artery (▶ Fig. 3.51). Embolization was performed utilizing Nester coils (Cook Medical, Bloomington, IN, USA): seven 4 mm × 7 cm coils, five 3 mm × 7 cm coils, two 6 mm × 7 cm coils, as well as one 2 mm × 4 cm detachable Ruby coil (Penumbra, Alameda, CA, USA) until hemostasis was achieved. The patient was successfully managed with coil embolization of the vessels feeding the pseudoaneurysm. He remained alive with no local tumor progression in the ablation zone and outside the liver as of last follow-up 2 years post-MW ablation.

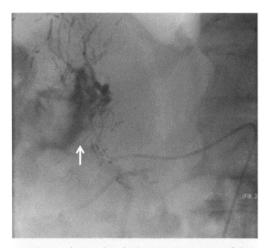

Fig. 3.51 Selective digital subtraction angiogram of the segment 4 hepatic artery displayed multifocal extravasation of contrast medium within the ablation zone (*arrow*). This was embolized with detachable metallic coils until complete hemostasis was reached.

Complication Analysis

Injury to adjacent vessels and bile ducts are rare but well-known complications of the thermal ablation. The goal of ablation with curative intent is to create margins of at least 5 mm, and ideally 10 mm circumferentially around the target tumor. This patient presented with a relatively large liver lesion (> 3 cm) in a challenging location, these factors increased risk of complications following MW ablation. Although the patient's complications were successfully managed and the patient was alive on last follow-up 2 years following initial treatment, the location was challenging and required special maneuvers. In such cases intra-arterial therapies including ^{90}Y radiation segmentectomy or DEBIRI TACE (beads loaded with 100 mg of irinotecan) could be considered instead of ablation, although the long-term outcomes of such therapies are not as well studied as with thermal ablation.

Strategies to Prevent and Take-Home Messages

- When treating secondary liver malignancies with a curative intent using percutaneous ablation, minimal ablation margins greater than 5 mm and ideally 10 mm circumferentially are necessary to achieve long-term local tumor control.
- Be aware of the potential increase in the complication risk when using thermal ablation (especially MW ablation) for large (> 3 cm) lesions, requiring multiple electrodes and overlapping ablations, especially in patient with prior hepatic artery infusion pump (HAIP) chemotherapy.
- [90]Y radiation segmentectomy or DEBIRI TACE could be considered instead of ablation for large lesions in challenging location, although the long-term outcomes of such therapies are not as well studied as with thermal ablation.

Further Reading

Liang P, Wang Y, Yu X, Dong B. Malignant liver tumors: treatment with percutaneous microwave ablation—complications among cohort of 1136 patients. Radiology. 2009; 251(3):933–940

Kwon HJ, Kim PN, Byun JH, et al. Various complications of percutaneous radiofrequency ablation for hepatic tumors: radiologic findings and technical tips. Acta Radiol. 2014; 55(9):1082–1092

3.2 Cement Extravasation

3.2.1 Pulmonary Cement Embolization after Vertebroplasty for Lumbar Fracture Treatment

Patient History

An 80-year-old male patient suffering from a single-level osteoporotic vertebral compression fracture (L3) and pain was scheduled for a minimal invasive treatment such as cementoplasty/vertebroplasty/kyphoplasty.

Initial Treatment

Transpedicular kyphoplasty lumbar 3. Prior angiography via needle placed in the vertebral body was done in order to evaluate run-off via paravertebral veins. The needle was placed in the mid-part of the vertebral body. Cement application was uneventful; the procedure was completed with a final fluoroscopy without any signs of mal-embolization.

Problems Encountered during the Treatment

No problems during the procedure were noted.

Imaging Plan

Routine chest imaging was scheduled 3 days after the procedure since the patient was suspected for pulmonary infection. Also, the upper part, mid-part, and also lower part of the right lung showed some opacification of distal pulmonary artery branches (▶ Fig. 3.52).

Resulting Complication

Embolization of cement during kyphoplasty which was done 3 days before.

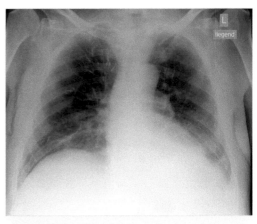

Fig. 3.52 Chest X-ray showing at the upper part, mid part and also lower part some opacification of distal pulmonary artery branches resulting from cement embolization during kyphoplasty.

What Would You Do?
Notes:
_____
_____
_____
_____
_____
_____
_____
_____

Possible Strategies for Complication Management

• Not available.

Final Complication Management

No treatment required.

Complication Analysis

Cement leakage is one of the major complications, which may cause severe consequence such as remote organ embolism or local chemical or compress symptoms. The polymethylmethacrylate could leak from the vertebral body deficiencies, fracture of the cortex, or through the vertebral venous system. Many previous reports also suggested vertebral body cortex fracture as a risk factor to cause cement leakage (CL). There are various factors that can effectively reduce the incidence of cement extravasation, including timing, injection volume, and so on. If treatment is delayed, leakage through a cortical defect is also less frequent. Unilateral percutaneous kyphoplasty (PKP) can reduce the risk of puncture and leakage than bilateral PKP. It can also easily control the needle position. It should be avoided to locate the needle position too near the crack of the cortical wall. High-viscosity cement is thought to be associated with low leakage rates and volumes.

Although preoperative CT scan should be used to detect cortical breakages depending on fracture location, the position of the needle should be adapted. The needle should usually be placed more anterior to avoid leakage to the canal when posterior wall breakage was detected. A broken posterior wall relates with higher rate of CL into the spinal canal. CL through endplate cortical disruption may be very quick and it can be hard to stop. Severe fracture and biconcave type both had higher leakage rate, as in these cases, it is very hard to drive the needle away from the cortical defects. However, most of the leakage incidents are symptomatic. Driving the needle away from the defect of vertebral body may provide some safety distance for cement spread and avoid leakage. Appropriate needle position could result in a safe place to inflate the balloon and consequently using high-viscosity cement could reduce leakage. However, cement could leak from several pathways.

Careful preoperative evaluation and using high-viscosity cement during the unilateral PKP procedure could prevent serious leakage and clinical symptoms. In the current case, low viscosity of cement and the effect of the paravertebral plexus were underestimated. However, this incidence was without any clinical sequelae for the patient and he recovered well since complete pain relieve was achieved.

Strategies to Prevent and Take-Home Message

- Perform angiography via lumbar needle to evaluate paravertebral vessel run-off.
- Evaluate CT scan for exact fracture location and try to achieve a needle position distant from the injured cortical wall.
- Check viscosity of cement before injecting.
- Try to stay with unilateral PKP.

Further Reading

Lin EP, Ekholm S, Hiwatashi A, Westesson PL. Vertebroplasty: cement leakage into the disc increases the risk of new fracture of adjacent vertebral body. AJNR Am J Neuroradiol. 2004; 25(2): 175–180

Walter J, Haciyakupoglu E, Waschke A, Kalff R, Ewald C. Cement leakage as a possible complication of balloon kyphoplasty—is there a difference between osteoporotic compression fractures (AO type A1) and incomplete burst fractures (AO type A3.1)? Acta Neurochir (Wien). 2012; 154(2):313–319

Nieuwenhuijse MJ, Van Erkel AR, Dijkstra PD. Cement leakage in percutaneous vertebroplasty for osteoporotic vertebral compression fractures: identification of risk factors. Spine J. 2011; 11(9):839–848

Yeom JS, Kim WJ, Choy WS, Lee CK, Chang BS, Kang JW. Leakage of cement in percutaneous transpedicular vertebroplasty for painful osteoporotic compression fractures. J Bone Joint Surg Br. 2003; 85(1):83–89

Ding J, Zhang Q, Zhu J, et al. Risk factors for predicting cement leakage following percutaneous vertebroplasty for osteoporotic vertebral compression fractures. Eur Spine J. 2016; 25(11): 3411–3417

3.2.2 Endplate Cement Extravasation after Balloon Kyphoplasty for Treatment of Osteoporotic Fracture

Patient History

A 72-year-old female patient with steroid-induced osteoporosis and several comorbidities (hypertension, coronary heart disease, diabetes, Basedow's disease, and rheumatoid arthritis) presented with painful compression fractures of the lumbar vertebrae 1 to 3. Malignancy was ruled out by biopsy (▶ Fig. 3.53).

Initial Treatment

Balloon kyphoplasty.

Problems Encountered during the Treatment

Compression deformity was corrected in all treated vertebra by balloon application. Fluoroscopy-guided cement-augmentation revealed endplate extravasations in the first and third vertebral bodies (▶ Fig. 3.54). Otherwise unremarkable procedure, no complications reported. Especially major complications, such as cement leakage into the spinal canal, neurologic compromise, embolisms to the aorta, vena cava, azygos vein, and the lungs were absent.

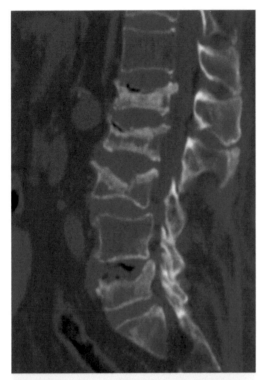

Fig. 3.53 Nonenhanced CT of the lumbar spine revealing the compression fractures of the lumbar vertebra 1–3 and 5.

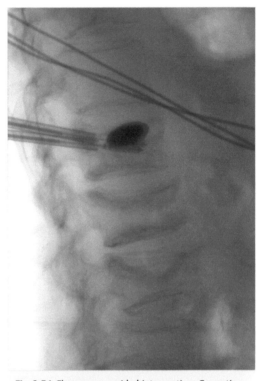

Fig. 3.54 Fluoroscopy-guided intervention. Correction of the compression deformity by balloon application.

Imaging Plan

CT, fluoroscopy, and MRI.

Resulting Complication

Intradiscal polymethylacrylate extravasation in two segments (▶ Fig. 3.55, ▶ Fig. 3.56, ▶ Fig. 3.57).

Possible Strategies for Complication Management

- Balloon kyphoplasty of the fractured adjacent vertebral bodies.
- Vertebroplasty of the fractured adjacent vertebral bodies.
- Surgery.

Final Complication Management

In case the pain persists despite the conventional medical therapy, further balloon kyphoplasty of the thoracic vertebrae 11 and 12 is projected.

Complication Analysis

Intradiscal cement extravasation resulted in an adjacent vertebral fracture.

Strategies to Prevent and Take-Home Message

- Cement application should be controlled under fluoroscopy.
- The use of the eggshell technique, including another balloon placement once the cement has been inserted in order to achieve a better distribution, may have potential to reduce the leakage rate.
- The most frequent complication following vertebroplasty and balloon kyphoplasty is the adjacent level fracture (41% in kyphoplasty and 30% in vertebroplasty). This is associated with cement endplate extravasation isolated to the anterior third of the vertebral body.

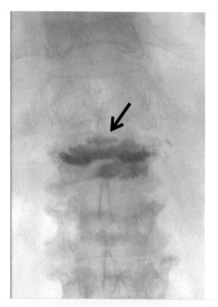

Fig. 3.55 Fluoroscopy indicates an endplate leakage with cement extravasation into the intradiscal space (*arrow*).

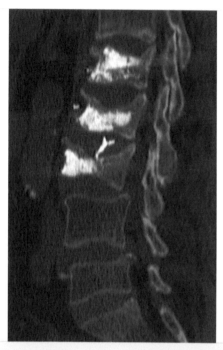

Fig. 3.56 Follow-up imaging in CT illustrate the cement extravasation into the anterior third of the intradiscal space in the first lumbar vertebra as well as into the middle third of the third lumbar vertebra.

Further Reading

Bergmann M, Oberkircher L, Bliemel C, Frangen TM, Ruchholtz S, Krüger A. Early clinical outcome and complications related to balloon kyphoplasty. Orthop Rev (Pavia). 2012; 4(2):e25

Jesse MK, Petersen, B, Glueck, D, Kriedler S. Effect of the location of endplate cement extravasation on adjacent level fracture in osteoporotic patients undergoing vertebroplasty and kyphoplasty. Pain Physician. 2015; 18(5):E805–E814

Ateş A, Gemalmaz HC, Deveci MA, Şimşek SA, Çetin E, Şenköylü A. Comparison of effectiveness of kyphoplasty and vertebroplasty in patients with osteoporotic vertebra fractures. Acta Orthop Traumatol Turc. 2016; 50(6):619–622

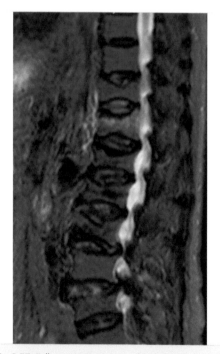

Fig. 3.57 Follow-up MRI 3 years after balloon kyphoplasty, revealing the acute compression fracture of the 12th thoracic vertebra.

3.2.3 Intra-articular Cement Leakage after Bone Augmentation in the Peripheral Skeleton

Patient History

A 54-year-old female patient with a medical record of breast carcinoma and diffuse metastatic disease including numerous bone lesions presents with pain and mobility impairment due to an osteolytic lesion located in the right femoral neck with a degree of cortical destruction. Among others, pain prevents the patient for undergoing radiotherapy for metastatic lesions in the spine (▶ Fig. 3.58).

Initial Treatment

Fluoroscopy-guided microwave ablation and percutaneous augmented osteoplasty under general anesthesia was performed. Under strict sterility, and fluoroscopy, two bone trocars were percutaneously introduced through the greater trochanter, following the natural lines of the Haversian canal system; both trocars were positioned inside the lesion. Coaxially, a 14G antenna was introduced and connected to a high power microwave generator system (140 W to 2,450 MHz). Ablation session characteristics: 40 W × 10 minutes. Following a metallic mesh of microneedles was placed inside the lesion and followed by polymethylmethacrylate injection ("rebar concept"; ▶ Fig. 3.59).

What Would You Do?

Notes:

_____

_____

_____

_____

_____

_____

_____

_____

Problems Encountered during the Treatment

Intra-articular cement leakage (▶ Fig. 3.60).

Imaging Plan

Follow-up with CT scan.

Resulting Complication

Intra-articular cement leakage: patient reports total pain relief when sitting or lying down; however, a new type of pain is present during walking.

Possible Strategies for Complication Management

- Immediate massage and mobilization of the joint.
- Intra-articular hyaluronate injection.
- Arthroscopic operation.
- Surgical operation.

Final Complication Management

Intra-articular cement leakage was verified during the injection process; immediate massage and joint mobilization were performed in order to dissolve the cement to smaller fragments. One week later due to complaints of the patient describing a new type of pain present during walking an intra-articular injection of hyaluronate solution was performed. Patient reported 60% pain reduction (▶ Fig. 3.61).

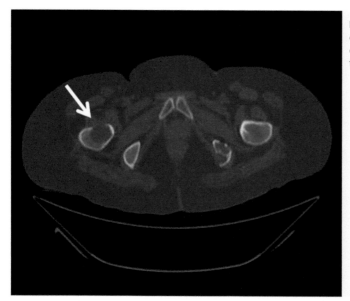

Fig. 3.58 CT axial scan illustrating the osteolytic lesion along with the cortical destruction (*arrow*) at the right femoral bone.

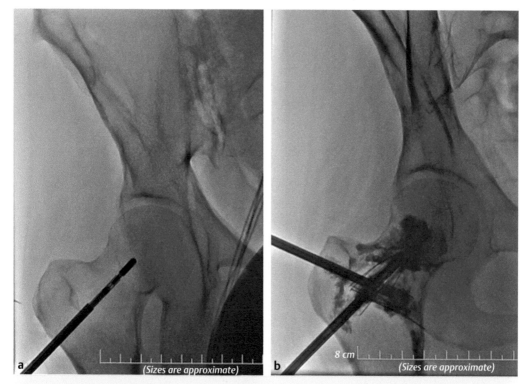

Fig. 3.59 Fluoroscopy views. **(a)** A 14G microwave antenna was introduced coaxially through the bone trocar and ablation session was performed (40 W × 10 minutes). **(b)** Two bone trocars were percutaneously introduced through the greater trochanter, following the natural lines of the Haversian canal system inside the lesion; a metallic mesh of microneedles was created inside the lesion and polymethylmethacrylate injection followed ("rebar concept").

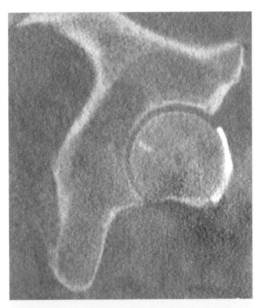

Fig. 3.60 Cone beam CT scan illustrating the intra-articular cement leakage.

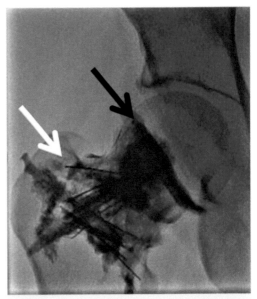

Fig. 3.61 Fluoroscopy view during intra-articular injection of hyaluronate solution; *white arrow* illustrates the needle used to gain intra-articular access—the *black arrow* illustrates the contrast medium injected to verify correct intra-articular location of the needle.

Complication Analysis

Due to cortical lysis, cement leakage inside the articulation occurred. The feared outcomes of such complication include potential chondrolysis along with a mechanical type of pain due to presence of cement intra-articular, which acts as a foreign body.

Strategies to Prevent and Take-Home Message

- Cortical lysis is a significant factor for cement leakage during cement injection in the peripheral skeleton.
- Cement injection should always be performed under continuous fluoroscopic control.
- In weight-bearing locations and specifically in long bones cement should be combined to some kind of instrumentation (cannulated screws, polymer or other metallic implants) for optimal stabilization and augmentation.

- In case of cement leakage inside an articulation, immediate massage and mobilization is warranted as an attempt to dissolve the cement to smaller fragments.
- Intra-articular injections of hyaluronate in such cases provide limited to moderate pain reduction and mobility improvement.

Further Reading

Kelekis A, Filippiadis D, Anselmetti G, et al. Percutaneous augmented peripheral osteoplasty in long bones of oncologic patients for pain reduction and prevention of impeding pathologic fracture: the rebar concept. Cardiovasc Intervent Radiol. 2016; 39(1):90–96

Cazzato RL, Buy X, Eker O, Fabre T, Palussiere J. Percutaneous long bone cementoplasty of the limbs: experience with fifty-one non-surgical patients. Eur Radiol. 2014; 24(12):3059–3068

Leclair A, Gangi A, Lacaze F, et al. Rapid chondrolysis after an intra-articular leak of bone cement in treatment of a benign acetabular subchondral cyst: an unusual complication of percutaneous injection of acrylic cement. Skeletal Radiol. 2000; 29(5): 275–278

3.3 Device Failure

3.3.1 Two Cases of Short Antenna during Microwave Ablation for Treatment of Lung Nodules

Patient History

Case 1: A 61-year-old male patient with incidental finding of a left upper lobe 12 mm pleural-based subsolid nodule (▸ Fig. 3.62a). Currently a smoker.

Initial Imaging and Treatment Plan

Due to the peripheral location of the small target lesion, CT-guided core biopsy was performed for tissue diagnosis (▸ Fig. 3.62); the patient was placed in right lateral decubitus position and CT-guided core biopsy was performed via a 10 cm 19G coaxial needle (▸ Fig. 3.62b), the histology revealing adenocarcinoma. FDG-PET scan showed no evidence of nodal or hematogenous metastatic spread.

In view of several comorbidities, the multidisciplinary team's joint decision was to treat the lesion with thermal ablation.

Owing to patient size and gantry confinements the decision was made to perform the ablation with the patient lying supine, choosing a left lateral pectoral access.

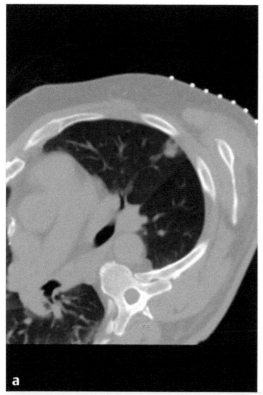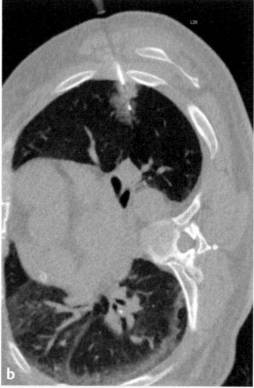

Fig. 3.62 CT-guided biopsy of left upper lobe lateral pleural based lesion **(a)** oblique position, planning grid on patient's skin **(b)** right lateral decubitus position; direct access chosen, coaxial needle in situ with tip just beyond the pleura and tip of the biopsy needle beyond the far edge of the target lesion.

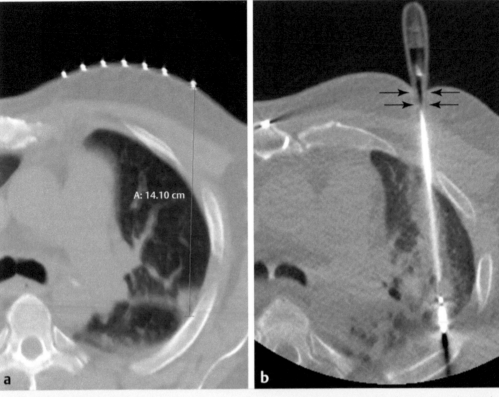

Fig. 3.63 CT-guided microwave ablation **(a)** supine position, planning grid on patient's skin; lateral pectoral vertical access chosen, total distance from skin surface to distal edge of the lesion was 14.10 cm **(b)** dependent atelectasis caused the target lesion to further fall back from the entry site, the microwave had to be actively pushed down, tenting the skin and indenting the subcutaneous fat tissue (*arrows*).

The measured distance between the skin and the distal edge of the target lesion was 14 cm (▶ Fig. 3.63a)—the length of the shaft of a standard Acculis pMTA microwave ablation antenna (Angiodynamics, Amsterdam, The Netherlands).

Problems Encountered during the Treatment

Dependent atelectasis with moving the target lesion slightly more posteroinferiorly lead to an increase of skin lesion distance.

In order to appropriately place the antenna with the feed point centrally within the target lesion, the antenna handle had to be forced into the subcutaneous tissue (▶ Fig. 3.63b).

Resulting Complication

No acute consequence other than the necessity to actively hold the antenna down throughout the ablation cycle.

What Would You Do?

Notes:

_____

_____

_____

_____

_____

_____

_____

_____

Possible Strategies for Complication Management

Reevaluate circumstances immediately before performing the procedure; allow for several centimeter leeway if possible. In the given example, the package with the ablation kit should not have been opened before the local anesthetic was administered and the target lesion was confirmed in its final position.

The case below illustrates a similar situation with a mobile target lesion:

Case 2: A 71-year-old male with a history of prostatectomy and pelvic lymph node dissection 7 years prior followed by salvage radiotherapy to pelvis; rising PSA indicated biochemical recurrence of prostate cancer; Ga-68 prostate specific membrane antigen PET/CT scan showed a solitary avid left apicoposterior subpleural lung nodule (▶ Fig. 3.64b).

The biopsy was performed with the patient lying prone, the mobile target lesion moved from one edge of the lung to the contralateral edge within the lung apex (▶ Fig. 3.65a). A pneumothorax occurred upon advancement of the coaxial needle—a 15 cm needle with a 10 cm shaft was chosen—displacing the nodule even further away from the entry site (▶ Fig. 3.65b).

The entire coaxial needle length was required to be advanced into the thoracic cavity to reach the displaced target lesion and allow for a successful core biopsy with a 2 cm throw (▶ Fig. 3.66).

Strategies to Prevent and Take-Home Message

When choosing the length of a biopsy needle or ablation device, consider that the final setup might differ from the planning, owing to many possible reasons—different position of the patient on the CT table, different suitable intercostal entry site, displacement of the target lesion due to change of position, atelectasis, or pneumothorax.

The equipment should not be unpacked until the final position for the intervention has been reached and verified.

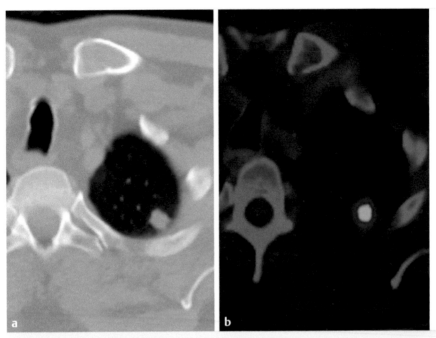

Fig. 3.64 Left apicoposterior nodule **(a)** axial CT scan, lung window **(b)** prostate-specific membrane antigen PET/CT scan showing avid left apicoposterior nodule.

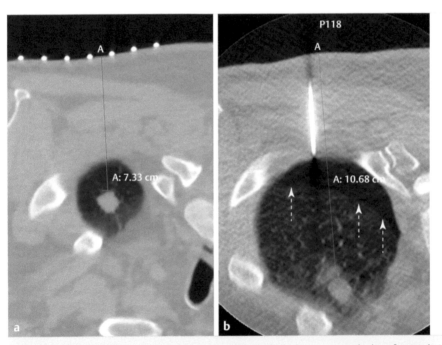

Fig. 3.65 (a) Prone position, planning grid on skin; distance from skin to proximal edge of target lesion 7.33 cm **(b)** coaxial needle in place, pneumothorax (*arrows*); the nodule has been displaced anteriorly and inferiorly, increasing the skin-to-lesion distance to 10.68 cm.

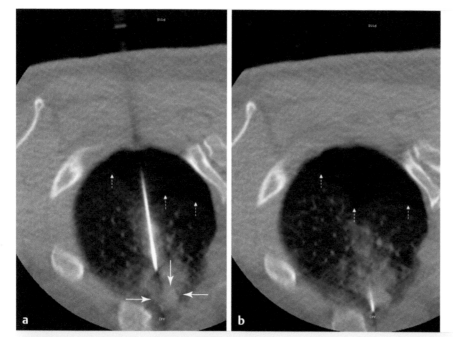

Fig. 3.66 CT-guided biopsy of left apicoposterior nodule **(a)** coaxial needle fully inserted, tip of the needle few mm short of the proximal edge of target lesion (*arrows*); minor hemorrhage along the needle and in perilesional distribution **(b)** biopsy needle with 2 cm throw passing through the lateral part of target lesion, which is now resting against the opposite part of the thoracic cavity. Note the pneumothorax in both images (*dotted arrows*).

Further Reading

Splatt AM, Steinke K. Major complications of high-energy micro-wave ablation for percutaneous CT-guided treatment of lung malignancies: Single-centre experience after 4 years. J Med Imaging Radiat Oncol. 2015;59(5):609–316

Cheng M, Fay M, Steinke K. Percutaneous CT-guided thermal abla-tion as salvage therapy for recurrent non-small cell lung cancer after external beam radiotherapy: A retrospective study. Int J Hyperthermia. 2016;32(3):316–323

3.3.2 Antenna Fracture during Microwave Ablation for Treatment of Non-small-Cell Lung Cancer

Patient History

This 88-year-old male, ex-smoker, was admitted to hospital for periprosthetic tibial fracture. His pre-operative chest X-ray showed an incidental left basal lung lesion, verified on subsequent CT imag-ing, FDG-PET avid. Biopsy revealed non-small-cell lung cancer. No nodal or distant metastases were present. Thermal ablation was considered the adequate treatment option.

Initial Imaging and Treatment Plan

An oblique access was chosen to allow the antenna to be introduced along the long axis of the tumor

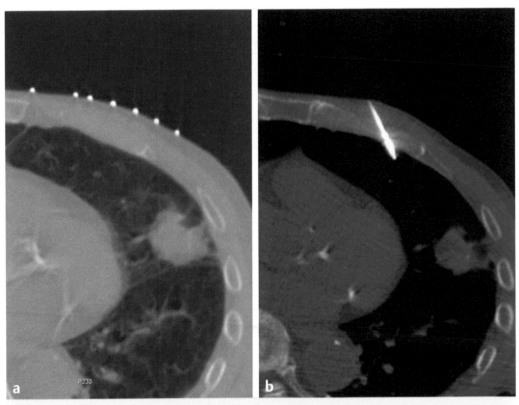

Fig. 3.67 Axial CT **(a)** lung window shows the planning scan, the 2.8 cm lobulated left upper lobe nodule abutting the oblique fissure **(b)** microwave antenna passing through costochondral cartilage.

and to avoid crossing the adjacent oblique fissure (▶ Fig. 3.67).

The introduction of the microwave antenna (standard 1.8 mm Accu2i pMTA applicator, Angio-Dynamics, Latham, NY, USA) required reasonable force while passing through the chest wall. Owing to the unusual shape of the antenna tip on the control scan and the slightly curved shaft with the tip of the antenna pointing toward the heart (▶ Fig. 3.68a) with inability to change direction due to the cartilage dictating the path, the decision was made to withdraw the antenna and appropriately reinsert.

Resulting Complication

The antenna was bent and the ceramic tip was missing. Repeat imaging showed the degloved ceramic tip lying anteriorly in the pleural space at the antenna entry site; a small pneumothorax had developed (▶ Fig. 3.68b).

Possible Strategies for Complication Management

- Abort and reschedule for thermal ablation.
- Abort and refer for thoracoscopy and ceramic tip retrieval.
- Continue with planned ablation using new antenna.

Final Complication Management

A 14-gauge coaxial needle was placed through the chest wall; however, the attempt to introduce a new antenna through the coaxial needle was unsuccessful owing to the sticky properties of the antenna coating. Despite this, the coaxial needle created a channel through the cartilage wide enough to allow for a new antenna (▶ Fig. 3.68b) to be subsequently inserted without major resistance and the ablation was performed as planned.

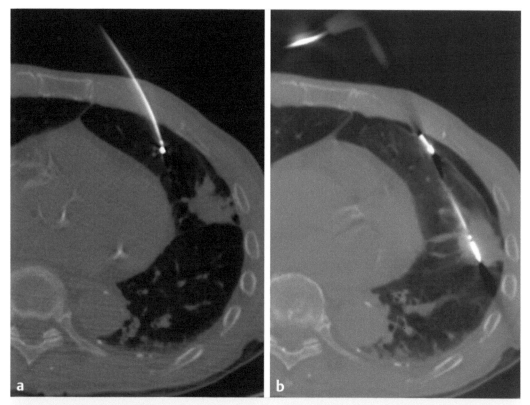

Fig. 3.68 Axial CT **(a)** intermediate window shows the bent antenna shaft and the distorted tip **(b)** ceramic tip lying in the pleural space, small pneumothorax and second microwave antenna introduced through the same access appropriately positioned within the target lesion.

▶ Fig. 3.69 shows the antenna with the broken tip and missing ceramic tip next to an undamaged antenna.

The manufacturer confirmed inert material of the ceramic tip, which was deemed safe to be left in place, especially in view of the fact that the tip caused no symptoms, and monitored with regular follow-up imaging.

The 3-hour chest X-ray showed focally enlarging pneumothorax and the ceramic tip projected over the descending aorta, between the hilum and the left heart border (▶ Fig. 3.70a). Enlarging pneumo-thorax led to the insertion of a pigtail catheter. A chest X-ray prior to pigtail catheter removal showed ceramic tip projected onto left paraverte-bral region level L1 (▶ Fig. 3.70b).

A CT scan 1 week later confirmed the location of the ceramic tip in the left pleural space, medially in the posterior costophrenic angle (▶ Fig. 3.71a). The patient had still no procedure-related symptoms. The position of the ceramic tip in 18 months had not changed (▶ Fig. 3.71b).

Complication Analysis, Strategies to Prevent, and Take-Home Message

In contrast to coaxial needles, biopsy needles and most radiofrequency ablation electrodes, micro-wave ablation antennae are not to be subjected to axial forces or to be inserted through rigid tissue such as cartilage or (calcified) pleural plaques.

If no alternative route is deemed safe and appro-priate, insertion of a coaxial needle is recom-mended and the antenna is introduced through the coaxial needle. Compatibility of coaxial needle and antenna should be ensured beforehand, as matching size (e.g., 14G coaxial needle and 15G antenna, as in the presented case), especially with products from different vendors, is not a guarantee for compatibility.

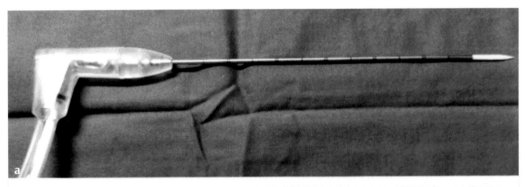

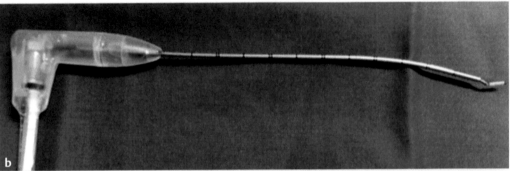

Fig. 3.69 **(a)** Undamaged standard 1.8 mm Accu2i pMTA microwave antenna. **(b)** Antenna with bent shaft, broken distorted tip, and missing ceramic tip component.

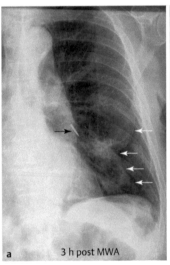

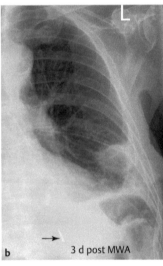

Fig. 3.70 Chest X-ray erect anteroposterior projection **(a)** 3 hours postablation; focal pneumothorax laterobasally (*white arrows*) adjacent to the target lesion, ceramic antenna tip (*black arrow*) **(b)** 3 days postablation, after removal of pigtail catheter from left pleural space; ceramic tip has migrated inferiorly, in the left paravertebral tissues level L1 (*arrow*).

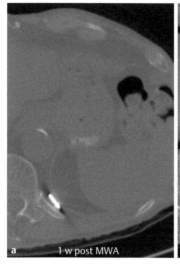
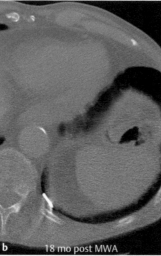

a 1 w post MWA b 18 mo post MWA

Fig. 3.71 Axial chest CT intermediate window **(a)** 1 week postablation; ceramic tip lies medially at left posterior costophrenic angle **(b)** 18 months postablation; position of ceramic tip unchanged, left lower lobe better ventilated.

Further Reading

Danaher LA, Steinke K. Hot tips on hot tips: technical problems with percutaneous insertion of a microwave antenna through rigid tissue. J Med Imaging Radiat Oncol. 2013; 57(1):57–60

3.3.3 Thermal Ablation: Cutting Off the Leg of a Radiofrequency Ablation Device during a Simultaneous Biopsy

Patient History

A 70-year-old female patient presents with retroperitoneal metastases of a renal cancer (coincidence of a clear cell renal cell carcinoma and a malign fibrous histiocytoma of the renal capsule, rated as a sarcoma). Histology revealed metastases of the sarcoma. Six years after surgery and adjuvant systemic chemotherapy with ifosfamide and adriamycin, a solitary liver metastasis appeared and was interdisciplinary decided to be treated locally. Histopathologic investigation should be performed to rule out an origin from the clear cell renal cell carcinoma.

Initial Treatment Received

CT-guided biopsy and radiofrequency ablation (▶ Fig. 3.72, ▶ Fig. 3.73).

Problems Encountered during the Treatment

In the absence of a coaxial system for biopsy and ablation, both devices were inserted parallel to each other. Taking one biopsy only, the umbrella-shaped radio frequency device was damaged and one leg was scissored during biopsy.

Imaging Plan

Nonenhanced CT.

Resulting Complication

The cropped leg of the radiofrequency device remained in the ablated target lesion (▶ Fig. 3.74).

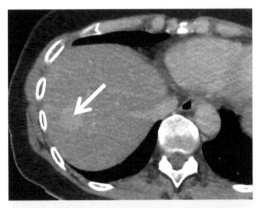

Fig. 3.72 Contrast-enhanced axial CT scan showing the target lesion (*arrow*).

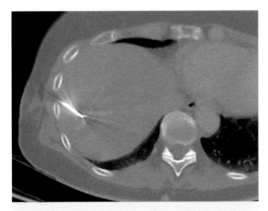

Fig. 3.73 CT-guided insertion of the radiofrequency device.

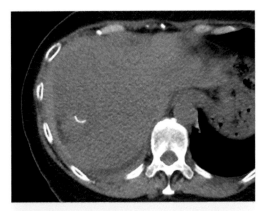

Fig. 3.74 Nonenhanced axial CT scan showing the cropped leg of the radiofrequency device; further a narrow capsular hematoma.

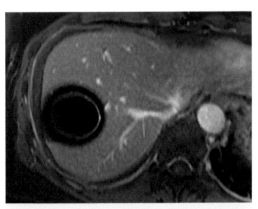

Fig. 3.75 Extensive signal extinction in MRI due to the ferromagnetic source of irritation.

Possible Strategies for Complication Management

- Follow-up imaging for exclusion of migration of the foreign body.
- Surgical removal.

Final Complication Management

Follow-up imaging was performed (▶ Fig. 3.75, ▶ Fig. 3.76).

Complication Analysis

Cropping a piece of a radiofrequency device during a simultaneous biopsy.

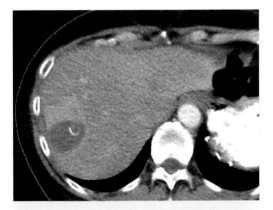

Fig. 3.76 Follow-up contrast-enhanced axial CT scan showing a complete ablation of the target lesion without malign remnant as well as a missing migration of the foreign body.

Strategies to Prevent and Take-Home Message

- Ensure that a coaxial device is available.
- Perform thermal ablation with a needle-shaped device, like a microwave probe.

Further Reading

Kim KR, Thomas S. Complications of image-guided thermal ablation of liver and kidney neoplasms. Semin Intervent Radiol. 2014; 31(2):138–148

Gillams A, Goldberg N, Ahmed M, et al. Thermal ablation of colorectal liver metastases: a position paper by an international panel of ablation experts, the Interventional Oncology Sans Frontières meeting 2013. Eur Radiol. 2015; 25(12):3438–3454

Su XF, Li N, Chen XF, Zhang L, Yan M. Incidence and risk factors for liver abscess after thermal ablation of liver neoplasm. Hepat Mon. 2016; 16(7):e34588

3.4 Infection

3.4.1 Hepatic Abscess after Transarterial Chemoembolization for Hepatocellular Carcinoma Treatment

Patient History

A 79-year-old male patient with infiltrative hepatocellular carcinoma (HCC) of the left hepatic lobe, previously treated with trans artererial radio embolization (TARE) and with progressive disease, was planned for transcatheter arterial embolization (TAE; ▶ Fig. 3.77a, b).

Initial Treatment

Catheterization of celiac trunk was performed with a 5F cobra catheter, demonstrating regular origin of the hepatic arteries and showing a slightly hypervascular mass (▶ Fig. 3.77c) supplied by the left and medium hepatic arteries. With a 3 French microcatheter 100 to 300μ beads (Embosphere, Merit Medical, Jordan, UT, USA) were administrated.

Problems Encountered during the Treatment

No acute complication; the patient was discharged the next day.

Imaging Plan

Routine follow-up with contrast-enhanced CT or MRI every month.

Resulting Complication

Ten days after the procedure the patient was admitted to the emergency room, with high fever, epigastric/mesogastric abdominal pain and leukocytosis (15,000/μL; normal values: 4,500–10,000/μL). An ultrasound examination was performed

▶ Fig. 3.78a–c) showing a liquid-corpusculated area in the left hepatic lobe in the hepatic territory treated with TAE (▶ Fig. 3.78c); a subsequent CT confirmed the presence of an inhomogeneous area with maximum diameter of 16 cm, air bubbles and enhancing borders (▶ Fig. 3.79).

The final diagnosis was hepatic abscess.

What Would You Do?

Notes:

_____

_____

_____

_____

_____

_____

_____

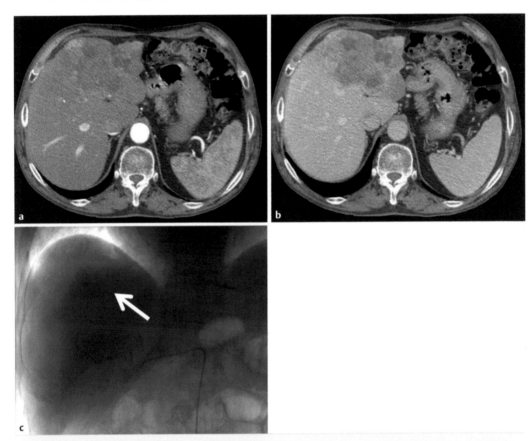

Fig. 3.77 CT scans **(a,b)** show a 13 × 9 cm infiltrative hepatocellular carcinoma lesion, occupying most of the left hepatic lobe; the mass only partially hyperdense in the arterial phase with hypodense appearance in subsequent phases. The slight hypervascularity of the mass is confirmed by the digital subtraction angiography image **(c)** obtained during the transcatheter arterial embolization procedure. Note the presence of coils, due to a previous transarterial radioembolization procedure (*arrow*).

Possible Strategies for Complication Management

- Conservative treatment (antibiotics, surveillance).
- Percutaneous abscess drainage.
- Surgery.

Final Complication Management

Percutaneous treatment: ultrasound and X-ray-guided placement of a 10 French tube drainage in the necrotic-infected collection with a right sub-costal approach in a moderately sedated patient (▶ Fig. 3.80).

One month after the procedure, CT showed size reduction of the abscess (▶ Fig. 3.81).

Complication Analysis

TAE is widely used as treatment for large and unresectable HCC. Hepatic abscess is a quite rare complication, related to the extent of liver infarction/mass treated, less commonly to the diameter of the embolized artery and the caliber of the chosen particles. When abscess occurs, it is due to colonization of necrotic tumor from either enteric organisms or from bacteria introduced exogenously during the procedure. Clinical management includes systemic antibiotic therapy for abscesses less than 5 cm and percutaneous drainage for larger loculated collections.

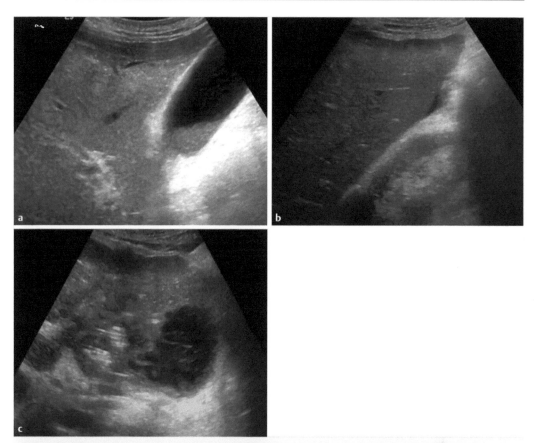

Fig. 3.78 Ultrasound images show gallbladder sludge **(a)**, fluid collection in the hepatorenal recess **(b)** and an inhomogeneous area **(c)** in the left hepatic lobe, medially to the one subjected to transcatheter arterial embolization.

Strategies to Prevent and Take-Home Message

Hepatic abscess is a rare complication after transarterial chemoembolization (TACE). Since an abscess is related to the extent of liver infarction/ mass treated more than to the diameter of the embolized artery and the caliber of the chosen particles, it is important to balance the procedure carefully in that manner, whether the entire mass should be treated within one session, or splitting in two or even more sessions is indicated. The larger the mass is, and the less healthy liver tissue covers the mass, the more care is warranted for TACE. Due to the fact that colonization of necrotic tumor results from either enteric organisms or from bacteria introduced exogenously during the procedure, the procedure needs to be performed under greatest care in terms of sterile conditions.

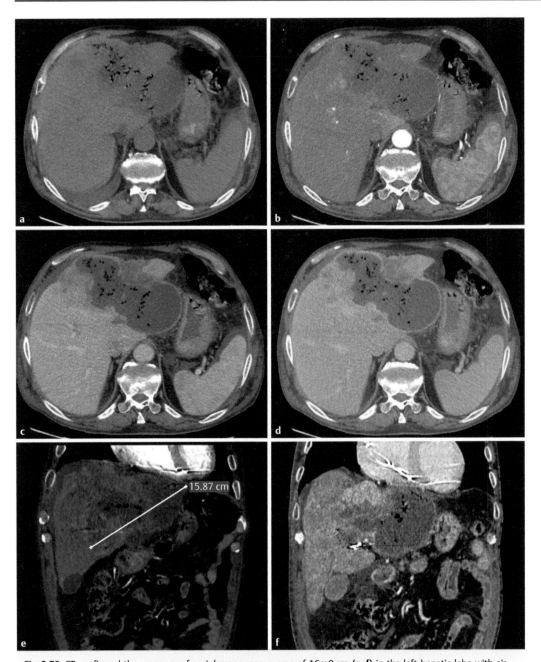

Fig. 3.79 CT confirmed the presence of an inhomogeneous area of 16 × 9 cm **(a–f)** in the left hepatic lobe with air bubbles within and enhancing borders **(a–d)**. Note the right subdiaphragmatic fluid collection **(a)**.

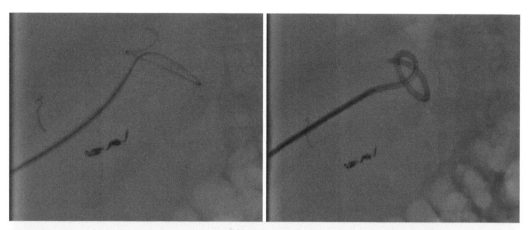

Fig. 3.80 X-ray images showing 10 French tube drainage placement with a right subcostal approach.

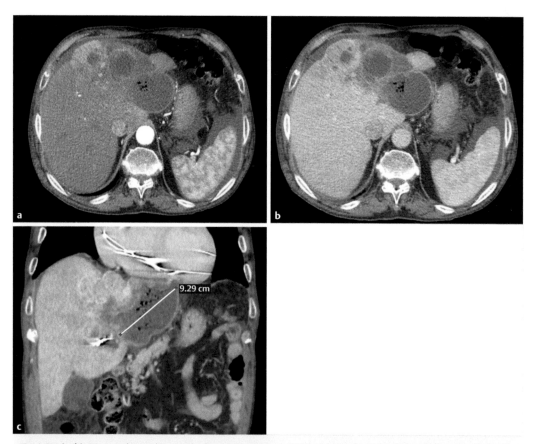

Fig. 3.81 (a, b) CT scan obtained 1 month after transcatheter arterial embolization procedure and drainage placement reveals abscess reduction (c), with larger diameter of 9.29 cm. Note the absence of the tube drainage, accidentally removed by the patient.

Further Reading

Vanderwalde AM, Marx H, Leong L. Liver abscess as a complication of hepatic transarterial chemoembolization: a case report, literature review, and clinical recommendations. Gastrointest Cancer Res. 2009; 3(6):247–251

Lv, WF, Lu, D, He, YS, Xiao, JK, Zhou, CZ, Cheng, DL. Liver abscess formation following transarterial chemoembolization. Medicine (Baltimore). 2016; 95(17):e3503

3.4.2 Liver Abscess after Transarterial Chemoembolization for Hepatocellular Carcinoma Treatment

Patient History

An 80-year-old male with recurrent hepatocellular carcinomas (HCCs) after left lobectomy was planned to undergo transarterial chemoembolization (TACE) for three HCC nodules. His performance status was good and his liver function was Child–Pugh A (score 6). Contrast-enhanced CT showed small hypervascular HCCs in the arterial phase (▶ Fig. 3.82).

Initial Treatment

A microcatheter was inserted into each feeding artery superselectively, and conventional TACE was carried out. Total 40 mg epidoxorubicin and 4 mL lipiodol was injected, and then, each feeding arteries were embolized with gelatin sponge particles. Plain CT just after the procedures showed good accumulation of lipiodol in each lesion (▶ Fig. 3.83).

Problems Encountered during the Treatment

None.

Imaging Plan

Routing imaging according to the institutional surveillance program.

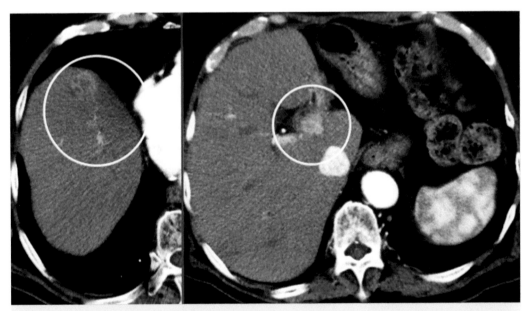

Fig. 3.82 Contrast-enhanced CT shows small hypervascular hepatocellular carcinoma lesions (*white circle*) in the arterial phase.

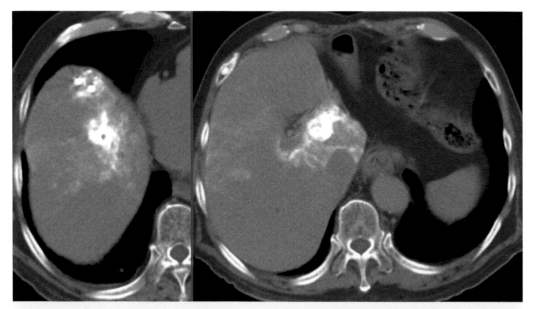

Fig. 3.83 CT just after superselective conventional transarterial chemoembolization procedure shows good lipoid accumulation in hepatocellular carcinoma lesions.

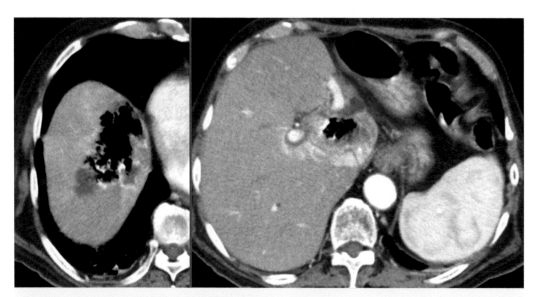

Fig. 3.84 Contrast-enhanced CT shows liver abscesses at the treated regions with conventional transarterial chemoembolization.

Resulting Complication

The spike fever occurred at the next day of conventional TACE procedure, and the increase of serum C-reactive protein was observed (29.7mg/dL).

Contrast-enhanced CT on day 5 revealed liver abscesses at the treated regions (► Fig. 3.84, ► Fig. 3.85).

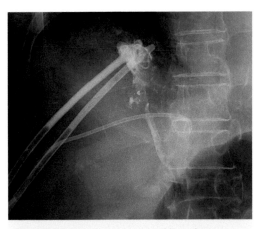

Fig. 3.85 Percutaneous drainages of liver abscesses were performed.

What Would You Do?

Notes:

_____

_____

_____

_____

_____

_____

_____

_____

Possible Strategies for Complication Management

- Continue drainage, until improvement is seen.
- Administer high dose antibiotics.
- Make the other drainage route.

Final Complication Management

Three drainage tubes were inserted to the liver abscesses percutaneously, and antibiotics were administered intravenously. Then, fever and blood–chemical data were significantly improved. One month later, the total drainage volume decreased to less than 10 mL/day, so the tube clamp tests were carried out to evaluate if the removal of tubes is possible or not. However, the fever occurred at the same day of tube clamp test, and it turned out that tubes could not be removed. We considered that the key point to remove percutaneous drainage tubes is to keep the drainage route. Therefore, we made a new drainage route connecting the abscess cavity to intrahepatic biliary system. We accessed biliary system percutaneously, and reached the abscess cavity via the biliary tree. Then, we put the biliary bare stent (Zilver stent 6 mm in diameter, 3 cm length, Cook Japan, Tokyo, Japan) bridging the abscess cavity and biliary system. After this procedure, the contrast injected into the abscess cavity smoothly flowed into the biliary system. Four days later, all drainage tubes were removed (▶ Fig. 3.86). (Two abscess cavities were already connected, and a tube of the remaining small abscess could be removed without the additional procedure.)

Complication Analysis

Liver abscess treatment after TACE is somewhat challenging, primary treatment option should be (selective) drainage placement.

Strategies to Prevent and Take-Home Message

In case of persistent liver abscess not allowing to remove the drainage tube, creating a connection between the abscess cavity and biliary system with a stent may be a considerable treatment option.

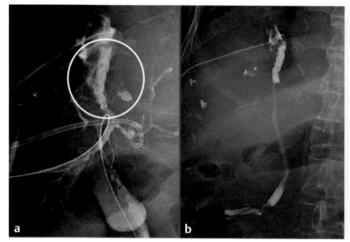

Fig. 3.86 With percutaneous access to the biliary system, biliary bare stent was inserted bridging the abscess cavity and biliary system (**a**, *circle*). Then, injected contrast into the abscess smoothly flows to biliary system through the stent (**b**).

Further Reading

Tu J, Jia Z, Ying X, et al. The incidence and outcome of major complication following conventional TAE/TACE for hepatocellular carcinoma. Medicine (Baltimore). 2016; 95(49):e5606

Lv WF, Lu D, He YS, Xiao JK, Zhou CZ, Cheng DL. Liver abscess formation following transarterial chemoembolization: clinical features, risk factors, bacteria spectrum, and percutaneous catheter drainage. Medicine (Baltimore). 2016; 95(17):e3503

Ikeda M, Arai Y, Park SJ, et al. Japan Interventional Radiology in Oncology Study Group (JIVROSG), Korea Interventional Radiology in Oncology Study Group (KIVROSG). Prospective study of transcatheter arterial chemoembolization for unresectable hepatocellular carcinoma: an Asian cooperative study between Japan and Korea. J Vasc Interv Radiol. 2013; 24(4):490–500

3.4.3 Injury of the Liver and Biliary System after Drug Eluting Beads Transcatheter Intra-arterial Chemoembolization

Patient History

A 52-year-old female patient who suffered from pancreatic cancer first received a pylorus-preserving pancreatoduodenectomy. After adjuvant chemotherapy with Gemcitabine, the disease progressed with diagnosis of multiple liver metastases 11 month after initial onset (▶ Fig. 3.87). Apart from a slight (glutamate pyruvate transaminase) GPT-elevation (61 U/l), liver function was nearly normal. Coagulation parameters were in standard range. The performance status was Eastern Cooperative Oncology Group (ECOG) 0. After the local tumor board reviewed the patient's case, an individual treatment of the liver metastases with transarterial chemoembolization (TACE) using irinotecan drug eluding beads was recommended while chemotherapy (systemic 5FU and oxaliplatin) was continued.

Initial Treatment

Following liver angiography (▶ Fig. 3.88) the patient received 3 mL DEB (drug eluting beads) in the size of 40 µg, loaded with 150 mg irinotecan in suspension with a contrast agent. Two-thirds of the dose was instilled in the right main liver artery and one-third in the left main liver artery until subtotal stasis in the liver arteries was achieved (▶ Fig. 3.89). The intervention was accompanied

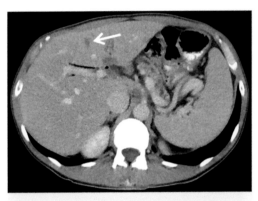

Fig. 3.87 CT before interventional treatment showing subtle pneumobilia after pylorus-preserving pancreatoduodenectomy, the portal vein is patent. Metastases visible in segment 4a (*arrow*).

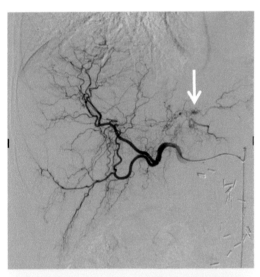

Fig. 3.88 Angiography prior to drug eluting beads transcatheter intraarterial chemoembolization showing the right branch of the main hepatic artery (*arrow*).

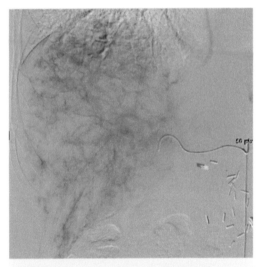

Fig. 3.89 Angiography after drug eluting beads transcatheter intraarterial chemoembolization showing stasis in the right hepatic artery.

by prophylactic antibiotic treatment with Ciprofloxacin.

Problems Encountered during the Treatment

Two days after DEB–TACE, the patient received a control CT (▶ Fig. 3.90) showing periportal edema. However, there was no evidence of postembolization syndrome (PES) with abdominal pain, nausea, vomiting, or fever. The patient was discharged

from hospital in stable condition two days after the intervention with antibiotic treatment; C-reactive protein (CRP) and GPT were slightly elevated.

Resulting Complication

Nine days after the procedure the patient was readmitted with clinical and laboratory signs of sepsis (RR 98/60 mm Hg, CRP 283.1 mg/L, temperature up to 41 °C). GPT/GOT have significantly increased (572/702 U/L). Abdominal contrast-enhanced CT (CECT) in portal venous phase showed large hypodense areas, mainly in the left liver lobe with entrapped air as well as evidence of peripheral portal vein thrombosis (▶ Fig. 3.91).

The patient was transferred to an intermediate care unit and treated with volume substitution and broad spectrum antibiotics.

The clinical status improved slowly while the infectious parameter decreased. Nevertheless, on day 18 after DEB–TACE the CECT showed an increase in size of the hypodense areas and an increase of the venous thrombosis (▶ Fig. 3.92).

Although cardiopulmonary status improved, the follow-up CECT 23 days after DEB–TACE showed further progression of the hypodense lesions involving the greater part of the liver parenchyma

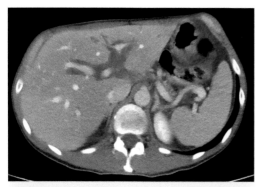

Fig. 3.90 CT 2 days after treatment showing periportal edema mainly left hepatic (CRP: 16.6 mg/L, GPT: 133 U/L, INR: 1.0).

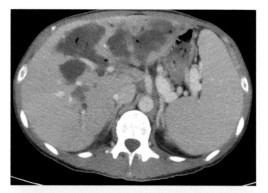

Fig. 3.91 Ten days after drug eluting beads transcatheter intraarterial chemoembolization: contrast-enhanced CT shows large hypodense areas mainly in the left lobe and presumably intraparenchymal gas (CRP: 284.9 mg/L, GPT: 572 U/L, INR: 1.3).

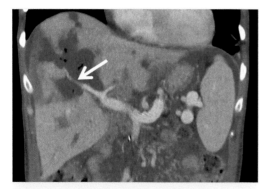

Fig. 3.92 Eighteen days after drug eluting beads transcatheter intraarterial chemoembolization: increased hypodense areas and progressive thrombosis of the right portal vein (*arrow*). Clinical status improved (CRP: 143.8 mg/L, GPT: 314 U/L, INR: 1.3).

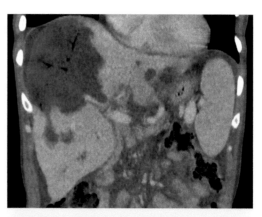

Fig. 3.93 Twenty-three days after drug eluting beads transcatheter intraarterial chemoembolization: subtotal necrosis of the partial left lobe and segments 7/8, complete thrombosis of the left portal vein. Nevertheless the patient was discharged from hospital in stable status (CRP: 193.7 mg/L, GPT: 367 U/L, INR: 1.2).

(▶ Fig. 3.93). However, due to clinical improvement, the patient was discharged from the hospital. At home, the patient became increasingly unstable with high elevated liver parameters and symptoms of liver failure. Additionally, a systemic inflammatory response syndrome occurred. Seven weeks after DEB–TACE the patient died as a result of gram-negative sepsis.

Complication Analysis

In the existing literature, the use of DEBs for TACE has several advantages, including better patient tolerability, deeper penetration of DEBs into to the tumor vascularization depending on small particle sizes, sustained, time-released delivery of chemotherapy into the tumor, as well as a significant reduction of the systemic plasma levels of the chemotherapeutic agents.

Clinically, the decreased exposure of systemic chemotherapy is correlated with fewer systemic side effects, such as nausea, vomiting, asthenia, and alopecia.

Despite the favorable safety profile, DEB–TACE is associated with increased locoregional hepatic toxicities compared to conventional TACE.

Since the beginning of local arterial hepatic therapies, there are reports about subsequent development of bile duct cysts, bile duct necrosis, and portal vein narrowing.

These adverse events were summarized to liver/biliary injury (LBI).

In 2012, Guiu et al described four types of liver/biliary injuries after DEB–TACE:

1. Intrahepatic bile duct dilatation.
2. Damage to the peribiliary plexus (PBP) with necrosis of the bile ducts due to decreased arterial blood flow or chemical insult of the vessel walls by the chemotherapeutic agent.
3. Portal venous thrombosis which might result from the collection of extravasated fluid in the Glisson capsule with compression of the portal vein branches; it may be related to an inflammatory process due to chemical vasculitis of the PBP.
4. Finally, biliomas result from necrosis of the bile duct due to ischemic/chemical insult of the PBP arteries whereas liver infarct requires concomitant arterial and portal vein occlusion.

Strategies to Prevent

In recent studies the occurrence of LBI after DEB–TACE was reported with a frequency of 30 to 36%. The treatment is usually symptomatic with antibiotics, volume substitution, and monitoring on the ward.

There seems to be no significant relationship between the type of tumor and the appearance of LBI.

However, it has been postulated that hypertrophy of the vascular peribiliary plexus in cirrhotic livers increases the development of vascular collateralization possibly resulting in a decreased risk for LBI in cirrhotic patients.

Since cirrhosis is a trigger for hepatocellular carcinoma (HCC) and about 50% of HCC patients suffer from cirrhosis, the risk of getting LBI seems to be lower in the treated HCC patients group.

Controversial data has been published regarding the influence of treatment selectivity and potential liver toxicities.

Until now, little is known about DEB–TACE-related locoregional toxicities; however, complications as cholecystitis and pleural effusion were reported to be more frequent with DEB–TACE performed nonselectively. Obviously, nonselective treatment exposes wider areas of nontumoral liver to potential toxicities. So far no significant association between the bead size and locoregional toxicities was found. However, in some single reports larger DEB size (> 300 μm) was held responsible for a higher rate of liver necrosis in patients with neuroendocrine tumors. There seems to be a relationship between the dose of chemotherapeutic agent and LBI; Monier demonstrated a correlation with higher concentrations of doxorubicin and the risk of LBI in HCC patients. Additionally, Monier discovered that a higher baseline prothrombin time (PT) value was significantly associated with biliary injuries, intrahepatic bilomas and global liver damage in HCC patients treated with DEB–TACE.

Take-Home Message

Locoregional complications occur in 30 to 36% after DEB–TACE. LBI represents a severe complication with probably fatal outcome. A selective or super selective access for the intra-arterial treatment should be chosen especially in noncirrhotic patients with elevated baseline PT values and dosage adjustment of the chemotherapeutic agent should be made.

Further Reading

Bester L, Meteling B, Boshell D, Chua TC, Morris DL. Transarterial chemoembolisation and radioembolisation for the treatment of primary liver cancer and secondary liver cancer: a review of literature. J Med Imaging Radiat Oncol. 2014; 58(3):341–352

Blackburn H, West S. Management of postembolization syndrome following hepatic transarterial chemoembolization for primary or metastatic liver cancer. Cancer Nurs. 2016; 39(5):E1–E18

Carter S, Martin Ii RC. Drug-eluting bead therapy in primary and metastatic disease of the liver. HPB (Oxford). 2009; 11(7):541–550

Greco G, Cascella T, Facciorusso A, et al. Transarterial chemoembolization using 40 μm drug eluting beads for hepatocellular carcinoma. World J Radiol. 2017; 9(5):245–252

Guiu B, Deschamps F, Aho S, et al. Liver/biliary injuries following chemoembolisation of endocrine tumours and hepatocellular carcinoma: lipiodol vs. drug-eluting beads. J Hepatol. 2012; 56 (3):609–617

Joskin J, de Baere T, Auperin A, et al. Predisposing factors of liver necrosis after transcatheter arterial chemoembolization in liver metastases from neuroendocrine tumor. Cardiovasc Intervent Radiol. 2015; 38(2):372–380

Lee S, Kim KM, Lee SJ, et al. Hepatic arterial damage after transarterial chemoembolization for the treatment of hepatocellular carcinoma: comparison of drug-eluting bead and conventional chemoembolization in a retrospective controlled study. Acta Radiol. 2017; 58(2):131–139

Martin R, Irurzun J, Munchart J, et al. Optimal technique and response of doxorubicin beads in hepatocellular cancer: bead size and dose. Korean J Hepatol. 2011; 17(1):51–60

Nicolini D, Svegliati-Baroni G, Candelari R, et al. Doxorubicin-eluting bead vs conventional transcatheter arterial chemoembolization for hepatocellular carcinoma before liver transplantation. World J Gastroenterol. 2013; 19(34):5622–5632

Odisio BC, Ashton A, Yan Y, et al. Transarterial hepatic chemoembolization with 70–150 μm drug-eluting beads: assessment of clinical safety and liver toxicity profile. J Vasc Interv Radiol. 2015; 26(7):965–971

Okuyama H, Ikeda M, Takahashi H, et al. Transarterial (chemo) embolization for liver metastases in patients with neuroendocrine tumors. Oncology. 2017; 92(6):353–359

Prajapati HJ, Xing M, Spivey JR, et al. Survival, efficacy, and safety of small versus large doxorubicin drug-eluting beads TACE chemoembolization in patients with unresectable HCC. AJR Am J Roentgenol. 2014; 203(6):W706–14

Richardson AJ, Laurence JM, Lam VW. Transarterial chemoembolization with irinotecan beads in the treatment of colorectal liver metastases: systematic review. J Vasc Interv Radiol. 2013; 24(8): 1209–1217

Rostas J, Tam A, Sato T, et al. Image-guided transarterial chemoembolization with drug-eluting beads loaded with doxorubicin (DEBDOX) for unresectable hepatic metastases from melanoma: technique and outcomes. Cardiovasc Intervent Radiol. 2017; 40 (9):1392–1400

Skowasch M, Schneider J, Otto G, et al. Midterm follow-up after DC-BEAD™-TACE of hepatocellular carcinoma (HCC). Eur J Radiol. 2012; 81(12):3857–3861

Toro A, Bertino G, Arcerito MC, et al. A lethal complication after transarterial chemoembolization with drug-eluting beads for hepatocellular carcinoma. Case Rep Surg. 2015; 2015:873601

Xie ZB, Wang XB, Peng YC, et al. Systematic review comparing the safety and efficacy of conventional and drug-eluting bead transarterial chemoembolization for inoperable hepatocellular carcinoma. Hepatol Res. 2015; 45(2):190–200

Marelli L, Stigliano R, Triantos C, et al. Transarterial therapy for hepatocellular carcinoma: which technique is more effective? A systematic review of cohort and randomized studies. Cardiovasc Intervent Radiol. 2007; 30(1):6–25

Lencioni R, de Baere T, Burrel M, et al. Transcatheter treatment of hepatocellular carcinoma with Doxorubicin-loaded DC Bead (DEBDOX): technical recommendations. Cardiovasc Intervent Radiol. 2012; 35(5):980–985

Monier A, Guiu B, Duran R, et al. Liver and biliary damages following transarterial chemoembolization of hepatocellular carcinoma: comparison between drug-eluting beads and lipiodol emulsion. Eur Radiol. 2017; 27(4):1431–1439

3.5 Non-vascular Miscellaneous Cases

3.5.1 Renal Defect after Cryoablation of Renal Tumor

Patient History

A 70-year-old female with left renal cell carcinoma (RCC) that was located in the upper pole of left kidney and 2.6 cm in diameter was treated with percutaneous cryoablation. The treatment was well completed without any complications.

Initial Treatment

With ultrasonography and CT guidance, the left RCC was treated with three cryoablation needles (Rod, Galil Medical Inc, Yokneam, Israel). Contrast-enhanced CT 3 months after the procedure showed the disappearance of enhancement of the tumor; however, the dilatation of left renal pelvis and ureter stone were also observed (▶ Fig. 3.94).

Problems Encountered during the Treatment

No problems during the procedure occurred.

Imaging Plan

Patient was scheduled for a routine follow-up with contrast-enhanced CT.

Resulting Complication

Four months after the procedure, the patient came back to the hospital because of left back pain. CT showed an urinoma around the upper pole of the left kidney (▶ Fig. 3.95), and that urine leakage coming out through the renal defect of cryoablated region was revealed.

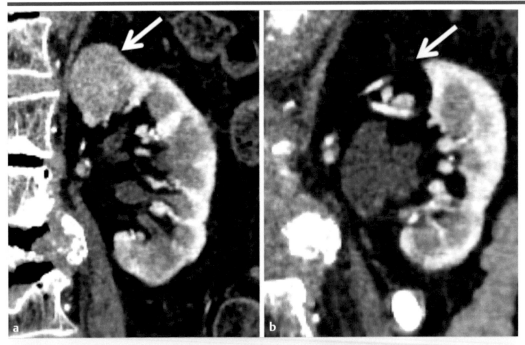

Fig. 3.94 Contrast-enhanced CT shows a renal cell carcinoma (*arrow*) in the upper pole of left kidney (**a**). Contrast-enhanced CT at 3 months after the cryoablation shows the disappearance of tumor enhancement (*arrow*), but also the dilatation of renal pelvis and ureter stone are observed (**b**).

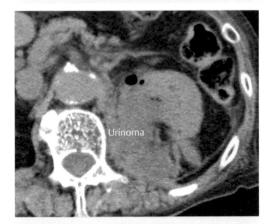

Fig. 3.95 CT shows the urinoma around the upper pole of left kidney.

What Would You Do?

Notes:

_____

_____

_____

_____

_____

_____

_____

_____

Possible Strategies for Complication Management

- Left nephrectomy.
- Stone removal and surgical repair of the renal defect.
- Stone removal and percutaneous closure of the renal defect.

Final Complication Management

At first, the left nephrostomy was made, and under the injection of contrast via the nephrostomy router, introducer system was inserted through the renal defect, and removal of the left ureter stone with basket devices was carried out through the renal defect. Then, through introducer system, two 0.035 inch guide wires (Cook Japan, Tokyo, Japan/Terumo, Tokyo, Japan) were inserted into the renal pelvis. Coaxially with a guide wire, 5 French angiographic occlusion balloon catheter was inserted, and the balloon was inflated in the renal pelvis. Coaxially with another guide wire, 6.5 French seeking catheter (Hanako Medical, Saitama, Japan) was inserted in to the renal defect. With pulling back the balloon catheter to avoid coil migration into the renal pelvis, 0.035 inch pushable coils (Cook Japan, Tokyo, Japan) were inserted into the renal defect using the 6.5 French seeking catheter. After dense packing of coils in the renal defect, the balloon was deflated and the balloon catheter was gently removed (▶ Fig. 3.96, ▶ Fig. 3.97, ▶ Fig. 3.98). Two days after the procedures, the nephrostomy tube was removed.

Complication Analysis

Tissue and tract defect after ablation might occur and should be detected by controlled surveillance program by imaging.

Strategies to Prevent and Take-Home Message

The tract or defect of kidney can be occluded with coils or other embolization devices if the migration of embolization devices into the renal pelvis can be avoided. The occlusion balloon catheter is helpful for this matter, and this technique can be used for not only the occlusion of a renal defect, but also for stopping the bleeding from the tract of nephrostomy and biopsy.

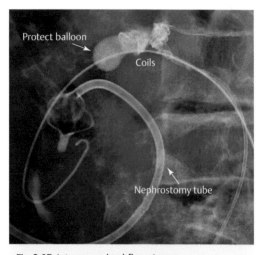

Fig. 3.97 Intra-procedural fluoroimage.

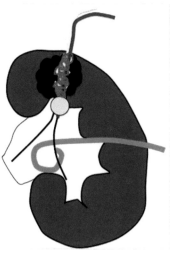

Fig. 3.96 Scheme of the defect occlusion with coils.

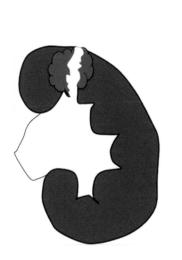

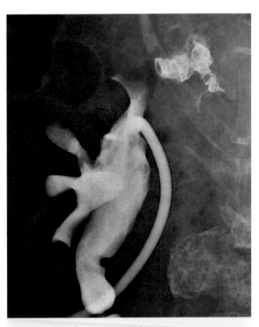

Fig. 3.98 The fluoroimage under contrast injection via the nephrostomy. No leakage of contrast from the renal defect is observed.

Further Reading

Blute ML, Jr, Okhunov Z, Moreira DM, et al. Image-guided percutaneous renal cryoablation: preoperative risk factors for recurrence and complications. BJU Int. 2013; 111 4 Pt B:E181–E185

Tokue H, Takeuchi Y, Arai Y, Tsushima Y, Endo K. Anchoring system-assisted coil tract embolization: a new technique for management of arterial bleeding associated with percutaneous nephrostomy. J Vasc Interv Radiol. 2011; 22(11):1625–1629

3.5.2 A Bronchial Fistula Following Percutaneous Lung Microwave Ablation

Patient History

A 58-year-old female patient with a previously resected kidney cancer was referred for management of a lung nodule of the left upper lobe (▶ Fig. 3.99). CT-guided lung biopsy confirmed metastatic nature of the nodule. The patient was oligometastatic, completely asymptomatic, and her ECOG (Eastern Cooperative Oncology Group) performance status was 0. Patient's medical treatment included only antiangiogenetic therapy for her primary kidney cancer.

Following the decision of a multidisciplinary tumor board, the patient was offered surgical resection or percutaneous CT-guided thermal ablation. The patient opted for the second alternative.

Initial Treatment

Due to the size of the target tumor (maximum diameter 28 mm) and the oligometastatic status

of the patient, percutaneous microwave ablation was chosen in order to maximize local tumor control. The antiangiogenetic therapy was discontinued before the procedure. Under general anesthesia and CT guidance, a 14-gauge microwave antenna (Amica HS, Latina, Italy) was deployed (▶ Fig. 3.100) inside the target tumor; and three different ablations were performed at the posteroinferior (40 W, 5 minutes), posterosuperior (40 W, 4 minutes), and anterior aspect (40 W, 4 minutes) of the tumor. The procedure was concluded uneventful, and a large ground-glass area abutting the homolateral hilum of the lung and the chest wall was noted around the target tumor (*dotted circle*, ▶ Fig. 3.101). The patient was completely asymptomatic, and thus, being discharged the day after the procedure. Antiangiogenetic therapy was immediately restarted.

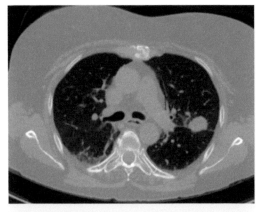

Fig. 3.99 Axial CT scan showing the target lung nodule of the left upper lobe.

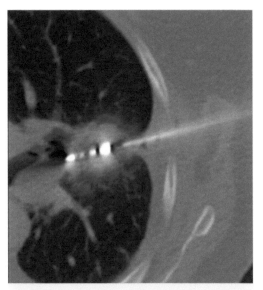

Fig. 3.100 The 14-gauge microwave antenna deployed inside the target tumor.

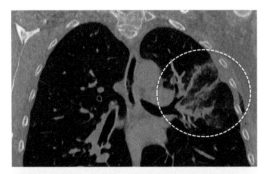

Fig. 3.101 A large ground-glass area (*dotted circle*) abutting the hilum of the lung and the chest wall was noted around the target tumor at the end of the procedure.

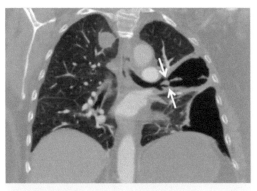

Fig. 3.102 Excavation of the ablation area communicating with two first-order bronchi (*arrows*); the homolateral pneumothorax is also seen at the base of the left lung.

Problems Encountered during the Treatment

None. However, 10 days later, the patient was readmitted to the hospital due to cough, expectoration, and dyspnoea. At the admission, the patient was afebrile and her vital parameters were: respiratory rate 14/minute; SatO$_2$ 84% (with oxygen 1 L/ minute); heart rate 88 bpm; blood pressure 150/ 100 mm Hg; temperature 39 °C; fasting glucose 2,11 g/l (HbA1c 11.3%).

Imaging Plan

CT scan.

Resulting Complication

CT scan revealed an excavation of the ablation area, which communicated with two first-order bronchi (▶ Fig. 3.102); a homolateral pneumothorax was also noted.

What Would You Do?

Notes:

_____

_____

_____

_____

_____

_____

_____

_____

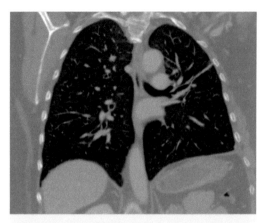

Fig. 3.103 Fibrotic healing of the cavity revealed at 12-month CT follow-up.

Possible Strategies for Complication Management

- Pneumectomy.
- Conservative treatment.

Final Complication Management

Despite pneumectomy was considered a possible therapeutic option, in accordance to literature, conservative management was adopted: antibiotic therapy was started and oxygen therapy continued until clinical conditions of the patient improved within 5 days from the admission; subsequently, the patient was discharged. Antibiotic therapy was continued for 6 weeks and patient underwent regular CT follow-up. Six-month CT scan showed a progressive retraction of the cavity, which completely healed 12-month after the procedure (▶ Fig. 3.103).

Complication Analysis

Cavitation is one of the possible evolutions of the ablation area following percutaneous lung tumor ablation. Factors predicting cavitation are target tumor near the chest wall, lung cancer as the primary tumor, and patients with pulmonary emphysema. Generally, cavitation evolves favorably and uneventfully although infection and abscess may occur, and should be suspected in case of inflammatory syndrome and/or radiological evidence of fluid levels inside the cavity. When cavitation communicates directly with a bronchus, a bronchial fistula is configured. A possible risk factor for bronchial fistula is a large area of ablation in proximity to a large caliber bronchus. Both these conditions were met in the present case since a large area of ablation resulting from three different impacts of the antenna was located in close proximity to the hilum of the lung. Moreover, other possible concurring factors in the present case may have been the early reintroduction of the antiangiogenetic therapy and the unknown decompensated diabetes since both these conditions can prevent or delay the fibrotic healing of the ablation area.

Strategies to Prevent and Take-Home Message

Clinically, bronchial fistulas present with cough, expectorations, and dyspnoea. Compared to an infected cavitation, bronchial fistulas rarely need an interventional management since expectoration through the concerned bronchus represents a natural way of drainage. For this reason, conservative management and regular CT follow-up are generally warranted until complete healing is noted on CT imaging.

Further Reading

Palussière J, Marcet B, Descat E, et al. Lung tumors treated with percutaneous radiofrequency ablation: computed tomography imaging follow-up. Cardiovasc Intervent Radiol. 2011; 34(5): 989–997

Okuma T, Matsuoka T, Yamamoto A, et al. Factors contributing to cavitation after CT-guided percutaneous radiofrequency ablation for lung tumors. J Vasc Interv Radiol. 2007; 18(3):399–404

Alberti N, Frulio N, Trillaud H, Jougon J, Jullie ML, Palussiere J. Pulmonary aspergilloma in a cavity formed after percutaneous radiofrequency ablation. Cardiovasc Intervent Radiol. 2014; 37 (2):537–540

Alberti N, Buy X, Frulio N, et al. Rare complications after lung percutaneous radiofrequency ablation: incidence, risk factors, prevention and management. Eur J Radiol. 2016; 85(6):1181–1191

3.5.3 Lethal Hepatocellular Tumor Rupture after Incomplete Chemoembolization: What Went Wrong?

Patient History

A 70-year-old male cirrhotic patient with history of chronic hepatitis C virus (HCV) infection that did not respond to interferon treatment, diabetes, arterial hypertension, and hypothyroidism was referred to our department for locoregional treatment of a focal lesion in the segment 6 of liver. The patient was affected by portal hypertension with the presence of large gastro-oesophageal varices combined with gastropathy, thrombocytopenia (50.000) but with relatively preserved synthetic function (INR 1.33, Bilirubin 1.44 mg/dL) and without signs of hepatic encephalopathy (model for end-stage liver disease [MELD] score 11). Patient was also receiving treatment with beta-blockers.

Imaging Plan

On ultrasound examination, a relative small nodular lesion in the lower hepatic edge was revealed; the value of alpha-fetoprotein was not elevated (1.86 ng/ml). CT imaging followed and confirmed the partially exophytic lesion in segment 6 with a maximum diameter of 3.8 cm and typical imaging characteristics for hepatocellular carcinoma (HCC) given also the background of the cirrhotic liver. The portal vein was patent and very limited amount of ascetic fluid was detected. CT-liver perfusion examination (GE-Revolution-GSI system, Cedex, France) also confirmed typical arterial blood flow elevation in the tumor nodule and no other intrahepatic or extrahepatic spread (▶ Fig. 3.104).

Initial Treatment

Transarterial Chemoembolization (TACE) Procedure was followed. After informed consent and having received antibiotic prophylaxis, patient underwent selective angiography followed by superselective catheterization of the sixth liver segment arterial branch with a 3 French microcatheter (Progreat, Terumo Interventional Systems, Somerset, NJ, USA). The tumor feeding branch could not be superselectively catheterized, so we decided first to advance the microcatheter to the nontumorous area and perform bland embolization of the healthy sixth segment with microspheres (75 μm) administration (Embozene, CeloNova BioSciences, San Antonio, USA). After that, we retrieved the catheter back to the main feeding branch and injected smaller (40 μm) microspheres (Tandem, CeloNova BioSciences, San Antonio, USA) loaded with 50 mg Doxorubicin Hydrochloride (Adriblastina, Pfizer Hellas, Athens, Greece) diluted with contrast medium up to a 5 mL volume After injection of the first 2 mL of the drug beads solution, contrast reflux was noted therefore injection was stopped. No contrast stagnation in the arterial branch was noted, however given the reflux the embolization was considered as complete and the catheter was withdrawn (▶ Fig. 3.105).

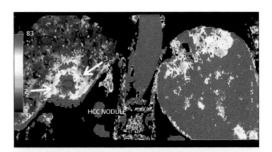

Fig. 3.104 CT–liver perfusion examination: "blood-flow parametric map" shows hypervascularization and typical arterial blood flow elevation inside the tumor nodule (*arrows*).

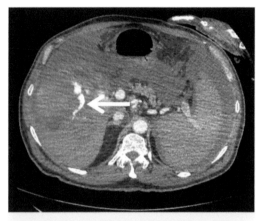

Fig. 3.106 Contrast-enhanced CT confirmed arterial extravasation (*arrow*) most probably from ruptured hepatocellular carcinoma. Intra-abdominal blood collections were detected in the perihepatic and the perisplenic spaces.

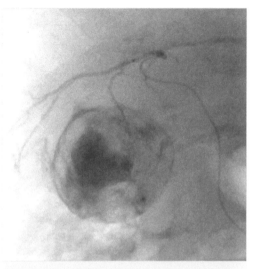

Fig. 3.105 Selective hepatic angiography confirms the hepatocellular carcinoma feeding branch toward the sixth liver segment. Despite incomplete contrast stagnation, chemoembolization was considered as successful.

Resulting Complication

Hepatocellular tumor rupture after incomplete chemoembolization.

Problems Encountered during the Treatment and Imaging Plan

The early hours after TACE, patient had an uncomplicated progress, with stable vital signs and only a mild abdominal discomfort and nausea that were relieved with standard treatment. Twelve hours after the procedure, patient developed hypotension without tachycardia (given the treatment beta-blocker) and a mild upper abdominal discomfort. The clinical evaluation was negative; no melena occurred and no signs of sepsis were detected. Nevertheless he received a fluid subtitution and the antibiotic regimen was upgraded to Piperacillin. Urgent blood tests showed roughly unchanged liver biochemistry with a small reduction in hemoglobin (~1.5 g/dL). Despite the initial response, the hemodynamic status of the patient did not improve and an urgent ultrasound was performed showing an extensive intraperitoneal fluid collection that was not present prior to the embolization, suggesting intraperitoneal bleeding. Subsequent tests confirmed severe decrease of the haematocrit, so patient was transfused with fresh frozen plasma and red blood cells. CT imaging with four contrast administration confirmed arterial bleeding, probably from ruptured HCC (▶ Fig. 3.106).

What Would You Do?

Notes:

_____

_____

_____

_____

_____

_____

_____

_____

Possible Strategies for Complication Management

- Conservative treatment for selected hemodynamically stable patients without evidence of active bleeding (blood replacement, correction of coagulopathy, cardiovascular monitoring).
- Emergency selective arterial embolization.
- Surgical procedures, such as liver resection and hemostatic procedures.

Final Complication Management

An urgent hepatic artery catheterization was performed revealing the diagnosis of rupture from a still patent HCC-feeding arterial branch (▶ Fig. 3.107). Immediate embolization with a 6 × 6.5 mm pushable coil (VortX, Boston Scientific, Marlborough, MA, USA) was performed and stopped the intraperitoneal extravazation (▶ Fig. 3.108). Unfortunately, the patient died 12 hours later due to multiorgan failure.

Complication Analysis

Spontaneous rupture of HCC is a fatal complication of advanced HCC, which is associated with high mortality rate. The risk factors associated with spontaneous rupture of HCC include large tumor size, capsular location of the tumor, contour protrusion, exophytic tumor growth, thrombosis of portal vein, and occlusion of feeding artery. Rupture of HCC after TACE is a life-threatening complication, which can cause severe bleeding and hypotension with increased mortality rate. The pathophysiologic mechanisms leading to spontaneous HCC rupture and HCC rupture following TACE are not fully known. It may be associated with tumor and capsular necrosis, vascular injury during TACE, inflammation from chemotherapeutic agents. Increased intratumoral pressure as a result of rapid edematic expansion after tumor necrosis may lead to HCC rupture. The peripheral location of the tumor, adjacent to the liver capsule is another significant risk factor for rupture.

Strategies to Prevent and Take-Home Message

- Large tumor size, location adjacent to the liver capsule, thrombosis of the portal venous system, and complete occlusion of the feeding artery are predisposing factors for HCC rupture after TACE. TACE should be avoided in patients with more than 50% tumor burden because of the strong association with rupture.
- Complete stasis should be the final stage after TACE, in order to prevent post-procedural bleeding from tumor rupture.

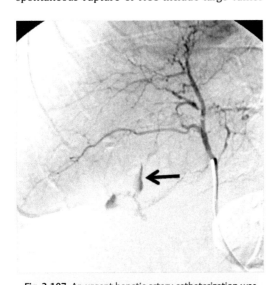

Fig. 3.107 An urgent hepatic artery catheterization was performed revealing diagnosis of intraperitoneal bleeding (*arrow*) from the still patent hepatocellular carcinoma feeding arterial branch.

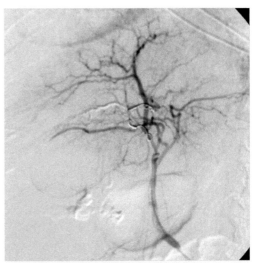

Fig. 3.108 Immediate embolization stopped intraperitoneal extravazation.

- The primary purpose of treating ruptured HCC is to achieve hemostasis by surgery, embolization, or conservative methods.
- Transarterial embolization is a feasible treatment option with high success rate for hemostasis and 30-day survival in patients with ruptured HCC.
- Patients with large amount of bleeding had poor prognosis despite successful embolization.

Further Reading

Lai EC, Lau WY. Spontaneous rupture of hepatocellular carcinoma: a systematic review. Arch Surg. 2006; 141(2):191–198

Cammà C, Schepis F, Orlando A, et al. Transarterial chemoembolization for unresectable hepatocellular carcinoma: meta-analysis of randomized controlled trials. Radiology. 2002; 224(1):47–54

Llovet JM, Bruix J. Systematic review of randomized trials for unresectable hepatocellular carcinoma: chemoembolization improves survival. Hepatology. 2003; 37(2):429–442

Brown DB, Nikolic B, Covey AM, et al. Society of Interventional Radiology Standards of Practice Committee. Quality improvement guidelines for transhepatic arterial chemoembolization, embolization, and chemotherapeutic infusion for hepatic malignancy. J Vasc Interv Radiol. 2012; 23(3):287–294

Xia J, Ren Z, Ye S, et al. Study of severe and rare complications of transarterial chemoembolization (TACE) for liver cancer. Eur J Radiol. 2006; 59(3):407–412

Zhu Q, Li J, Yan JJ, Huang L, Wu MC, Yan YQ. Predictors and clinical outcomes for spontaneous rupture of hepatocellular carcinoma. World J Gastroenterol. 2012; 18(48):7302–7307

Sun JH, Wang LG, Bao HW, et al. Emergency embolization in the treatment of ruptured hepatocellular carcinoma following transcatheter arterial chemoembolization. Hepatogastroenterology. 2010; 57(99–100):616–619

Jia Z, Tian F, Jiang G. Ruptured hepatic carcinoma after transcatheter arterial chemoembolization. Curr Ther Res Clin Exp. 2013; 74:41–43

Kim JY, Lee JS, Oh DH, Yim YH, Lee HK. Transcatheter arterial chemoembolization confers survival benefit in patients with a spontaneously ruptured hepatocellular carcinoma. Eur J Gastroenterol Hepatol. 2012; 24(6):640–645

3.5.4 Interstitial Pneumonitis after Microwave Ablation for Metastatic Lesion Treatment

Patient History

A 65-year-old female patient with a medical record of colorectal carcinoma (operated 18 months before) presents with a metastatic lesion in the lower lobe of the left lung. The lesion has both a component located in lung parenchyma as well as an intrabronchial component. No further comorbidities are reported.

Initial Treatment

Under sedation, strict sterility measures and CT guidance microwave ablation (MWA) was performed using a high power microwave generator (140 W to 2,450 MHz) with a 14G antenna—three ablation sessions were performed each 40 W × 5 minutes (antenna was repositioned between each ablation session; ► Fig. 3.109).

Problems Encountered during the Treatment

Unremarkable procedure, no complications reported.

Imaging Plan

Regular follow-up with CT scan.

Resulting Complication

1 month post the ablation session patient presents with fever and abdominal pain; follow-up scan

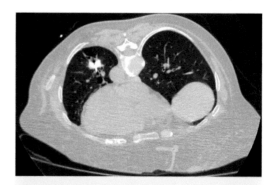

Fig. 3.109 CT axial scan during the microwave ablation session—patient is in prone position—the antenna is located close to the bronchus.

illustrates a thick walled cyst located at the ablation level and surrounded by extensive ground-glass infiltrate and minor pleural fluid collection (▶ Fig. 3.110).

What Would You Do?

Notes:

_____

_____

_____

_____

_____

_____

_____

_____

Possible Strategies for Complication Management

- Intravenous antibiosis.
- Percutaneous drainage.
- Surgical operation.

Final Complication Management

Patient was hospitalized for a week; intravenous antibiosis was administrated. Resolution of symptoms post 1 week antibiosis.

Complication Analysis

Extensive ablation zone produced by microwaves around and inside the bronchus resulted in cyst formation and postablation interstitial pneumonitis. Postintravenous antibiosis therapy a thin walled cyst remained regressing in size during the follow-up period (18 months; ▶ Fig. 3.111).

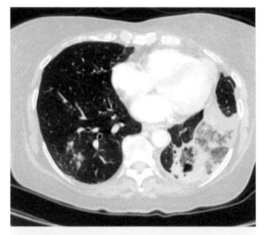

Fig. 3.110 CT axial scan at 1-month follow-up post the microwave ablation session—a thick walled cyst is located at the ablation level and surrounded by extensive ground-glass infiltrate along with minor pleural fluid collection.

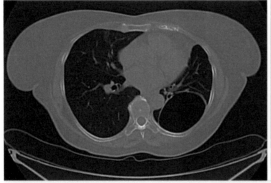 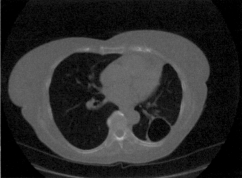

Fig. 3.111 CT axial scan during the follow-up period—a thin walled cyst remained regressing in size.

Strategies to Prevent and Take-Home Message

- MWA as compared to radiofrequency result in faster and larger ablation zones of higher temperatures since this kind of energy radiates through all biological tissues, including those with high impedance such as the air filled lung.
- Interstitial pneumonitis/pneumonia is associated to 0–25.0% mortality rate postradiotherapy, concerning postablation pneumonitis previous radiotherapy and age more than 65 years are considered risk factors.
- Tumor size of more than 3 cm in diameter and long-lasting procedures with multiple placements or repositions of the electrode or antenna may relate to lung abscess formation—it is advocated to minimize procedure time and electrode/antenna insertions during the ablation of large tumors.

Further Reading

Alberti N, Buy X, Frulio N, et al. Rare complications after lung percutaneous radiofrequency ablation: incidence, risk factors, prevention and management. Eur J Radiol. 2016; 85(6):1181–1191

Pereira PL, Masala S, Cardiovascular and Interventional Radiological Society of Europe (CIRSE). Standards of practice: guidelines for thermal ablation of primary and secondary lung tumors. Cardiovasc Intervent Radiol. 2012; 35(2):247–254

Kashima M, Yamakado K, Takaki H, et al. Complications after 1000 lung radiofrequency ablation sessions in 420 patients: a single center's experiences. AJR Am J Roentgenol. 2011; 197(4):W576–80

3.5.5 Insufficiency Fracture Following Bone Cryoablation

Patient History

A 76-year-old male patient with a previously resected esophageal cancer was referred for the management of a painful metastasis of the left iliac wing. The patient was painful both at rest and during daily activities (e.g., walking). Radiation therapy failed to achieve adequate pain control; therefore, the patient was referred for local treatment. A dedicated CT scan showed a large soft-tissue mass around the left iliac wing (▶ Fig. 3.112) coupled to an intense periosteal reaction.

Initial Treatment

Under general anesthesia, a percutaneous CT-guided cryoablation was performed by means of seven cryoprobes (5 Ice-Edge and 2 Ice-Rod; Galil Medical; Yokneam, Israel). A standard double-freezing protocol was applied to obtain a large ice-ball (▶ Fig. 3.113) completely encompassing the target tumor.

Problems Encountered during the Treatment

None. However, 1 month after cryoablation, the patient complained about the persistence of a mechanical pain while walking; no pain was reported at rest.

Imaging Plan

CT scan.

Resulting Complication

A bone insufficiency fracture (▶ Fig. 3.114) of the left iliac wing was noted at subsequent CT scan, thus, explaining the persistent mechanical pain.

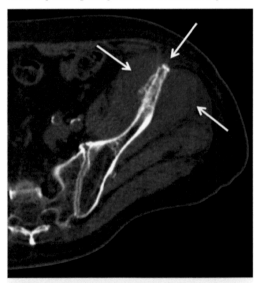

Fig. 3.112 Pretreatment CT scan showing the large soft-tissue mass around the left iliac wing (*arrows*) coupled to an intense periosteal reaction.

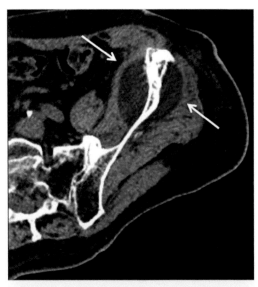

Fig. 3.113 The large hypodense iceball (*arrows*) encompassing the target tumor.

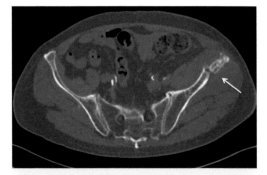

Fig. 3.114 Postablation insufficiency fracture (*arrow*) of the left iliac wing.

Possible Strategies for Complication Management

- Percutaneous cementoplasty.
- Percutaneous osteosynthesis.
- Surgical osteosynthesis.
- Conservative management.

Final Complication Management

Therefore, a percutaneous osteosynthesis was performed to fix the fracture under general anesthesia and combined CT/fluoroscopy guidance. The patient was installed supine; and three self-drilling cannulated screws (6.5 mm AsnisTM III Cannulated Screw System, Kalamazoo, MI, USA) were deployed coaxially over a metallic guidewire according to a previously described technique (reference N.1; ▶ Fig. 3.115). Additional cemeontoplasty was performed around the proximal part of the screws to increase their stability inside the bone in order to minimize the risk of loosening (▶ Fig. 3.116); in facts, at this level bone was considered brittle due to the primary disease and the subsequent cryoablation.

At 2-month clinical follow-up, the patient was completely pain free.

Complication Analysis

Bone metastatic disease affects up to 50% of cancer patients; and incidence is progressively increasing as overall survival of the oncologic population is progressively improving.

Bone metastases may be symptomatic in cases of: (1) bone insufficiency fractures secondary to chemotherapy, steroid treatment, radiation

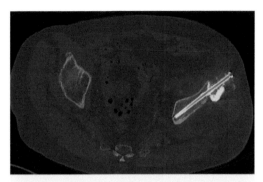

Fig. 3.115 Percutaneous osteosynthesis performed to fix the insufficiency fracture of the left iliac wing.

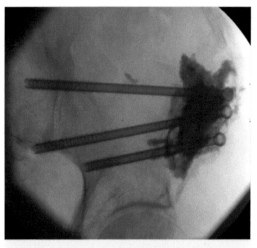

Fig. 3.116 Additional cemeontoplasty around the proximal part of the screws was performed along with osteosynthesis in order to increase screws stability inside the bone and to minimize the risk of loosening.

therapy, or percutaneous ablation; (2) pathological fractures secondary to bone replacement by tumor tissue; (3) impending fractures consistent with extensive tumor involvement of weight-bearing bones.

All these conditions may significantly affect patients' prognosis and quality of life due to pain, and increased morbidity and mortality. Therefore, therapeutic or prophylactic consolidation is warranted.

Bone insufficiency fractures occur due to osteopenia induced by chemotherapy or steroid treatment, or following local treatments (e.g., radiation therapy, percutaneous ablation) that weaken bone due to necrotic changes, and impair blood flow thus preventing adequate healing. Therefore, following percutaneous ablation, bone consolidation is warranted especially in highly solicited bones, in order to prevent secondary bone insufficiency fractures.

Consolidative treatments should be chosen based on the biomechanics of the target bone. In particular, where compressive forces are predominant (e.g., vertebral body, acetabulum, etc.) cementoplasty alone can be proposed. On the other, in areas where forces other than compression are involved (e.g., pelvic ring, femoral neck, etc.) screws mediated osteosynthesis may be proposed alone or in association to cementoplasty. In particular, cementoplasty can be added to osteosynthesis to minimize screws loosening or to fill a bone defect in case of pathologic or impending fractures.

Strategies to Prevent and Take-Home Message

Following percutaneous ablation, bone consolidation is warranted especially in highly solicited bones, to prevent secondary bone insufficiency fractures. Consolidative treatments should be chosen based on the biomechanics of the target bone.

Further Reading

Cazzato RL, Koch G, Buy X, et al. Percutaneous image-guided screw fixation of bone lesions in cancer patients: double-centre analysis of outcomes including local evolution of the treated focus. Cardiovasc Intervent Radiol. 2016; 39(10):1455–1463

Coleman RE. Clinical features of metastatic bone disease and risk of skeletal morbidity. Clin Cancer Res. 2006; 12(20 Pt 2):6243s–6249s

Manglani HH, Marco RA, Picciolo A, Healey JH. Orthopedic emergencies in cancer patients. Semin Oncol. 2000; 27(3):299–310

Cazzato RL, Buy X, Grasso RF, et al. Interventional radiologist's perspective on the management of bone metastatic disease. Eur J Surg Oncol. 2015; 41(8):967–974

Garnon J, Koch G, Ramamurthy N, et al. Percutaneous CT and fluoroscopy-guided screw fixation of pathological fractures in the shoulder girdle: technical report of 3 cases. Cardiovasc Intervent Radiol. 2016; 39(9):1332–1338

Cazzato RL, Garnon J, Tsoumakidou G, et al. Percutaneous image-guided screws mediated osteosynthesis of impeding and pathological/insufficiency fractures of the femoral neck in nonsurgical cancer patients. Eur J Radiol. 2017; 90:1–5

3.5.6 Postablation Biloma with Further Sequelae after Percutaneous Microwave Ablation for Treatment of Recurrent Metastasis

Patient History

A 51-year-old woman with rectal adenocarcinoma presented with recurrent metastasis posthepatectomy. She underwent biopsy and MWA of solitary FDG-avid recurrent 1.2 × 1.2 cm metastasis at the surgical biloma/resection margin in segments 2 or 3 of the remnant hemiliver.

The patient had a history of partial right hepatectomy, neoadjuvant chemoradiotherapy, and three prior systemic chemotherapy regimens including bevacizumab in addition to hepatic artery infusion pump (HAIP) chemotherapy. A preexisting postsurgical biloma (11.6 × 9.5 cm in size) and secondary mild biliary dilatation were present at the preablation scan (▶ Fig. 3.117).

Initial Treatment

Preablation biopsy was positive for malignancy. MWA was performed in supine position under ultrasound, CT fluoroscopy, and split-dose ^{18}F-FDG PET/CT guidance, using two Neuwave ablation PR15 electrodes (Ethicon, Madison, WI, USA) and a temperature probe (Medtronic, Minneapolis, MN, USA; ▶ Fig. 3.118). A total of three overlapping ablations were performed: ablation of 65 W for 6 minutes with one electrode, ablation of 65 W for 10 minutes with two electrodes, and final ablation of 65 W for 10 minutes with one electrode. Temperature monitoring was performed at ablation margin (1 cm away from tumor) with ablation termination when temperature reached 70 °C.

Immediate postablation triple phase contrast-enhanced CT and split-dose (second acquisition) ^{18}F-FDG PET/CT were performed and showed no evidence of residual disease. The minimal ablation margin was more than 10 mm around the target tumor and the ablation zone measured 5 × 3.6 × 3 cm. Postablation biopsies were performed within investigational Institutional review board (IRB)-approved protocol with specimens obtained from the ablation zone center and ablation margin with no evidence of viable tumor.

Problems Encountered during the Treatment and Imaging Plan

MWA was successful with evidence of complete ablation with sufficient margins both by imaging and pathologic assessment. The patient had fever (38.2 °C) the next day that resolved. Patient was asymptomatic and scheduled for the standard postablation multiphase CT scan in 1 month, to be used as a new baseline imaging for future comparisons.

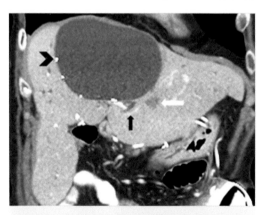

Fig. 3.117 Coronal, routine surveillance contrast-enhanced CT scan demonstrated a new hypodense tumor (*white arrow*). A large postsurgical biloma was again seen (*black arrowhead*). Biliary ductal dilatation in the left hepatic lobe was also seen (*black arrow*).

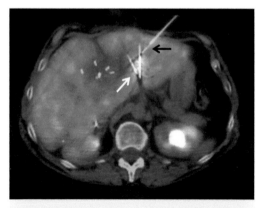

Fig. 3.118 Intra-procedural split-dose ^{18}F-FDG PET/CT scan was performed. Two NeuWave microwave PR 15 electrodes were placed within/around the tumor (*white arrow*), with a temperature sensing probe placed at the ideal margin of the tumor (10 mm from tumor) to verify appropriate marginal temperature was achieved (70 °C) (*black arrow*).

Resulting Complication

Nine days postablation patient presented with fever (39.4 °C), chills, abdominal pain, hypotension, and leucocytosis; contrast-enhanced CT scan revealed foci of gas within the 6 × 4 cm low density ablation zone (▶ Fig. 3.119).

Possible Strategies for Complication Management

Post-procedure gas within the ablation cavity is a common finding. In asymptomatic patients, no intervention is required, with follow-up imaging typically demonstrating resolution of gas within the ablation zone. In patients who have undergone prior surgery, especially pancreaticoduodenectomy, the risk of infection is much greater and such collections should be treated immediately. In addition, a course of prophylactic antibiotics for up to 14 days after the ablation can be considered in these high-risk patients.

When a patient is symptomatic, especially in the presence of fever and leukocytosis, a gas and fluid containing collection should be considered an

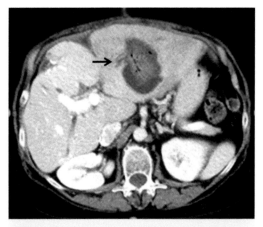

Fig. 3.119 Contrast-enhanced CT scan obtained when the patient became symptomatic (9 days after ablation). A hypodense ablation zone with foci of gas was seen (*arrow*), which could also represent normal postablation changes. However, this area was aspirated due to the patient's leucocytosis and fever, which raised concern for possible suprainfection. There was a minimal biliary ductal dilatation.

abscess until proven otherwise. Treatment should include the administration of a broad spectrum intravenous antibiotic and urgent drainage of the collection.

A connection to the biliary system can be recognized initially by observing the content of the fluid aspirated/draining from the collection. When bile drainage is suspected, the catheter should be interrogated with a contrast medium injection under fluoroscopy guidance to identify the damaged biliary duct and connection to the biliary tree. This connection may not be apparent when the collection is large or undergoing acute infection/inflammatory changes. Once the connection is identified, every attempt should be made to access the biliary system to divert the bile and facilitate healing.

Final Complication Management

Patient underwent CT-guided aspiration of the postablation hepatic collection, using a 20-gauge Wescott needle. It was exchanged for a 5 French catheter that was used to aspirate the fluid; this catheter was removed at the end of procedure. A total of 15 mL of turbid serous fluid was aspirated, nearly completely evacuating the collection, with sample sent to microbiology; culture was positive for gram-positive cocci. No additional fluid could be aspirated.

Microbiology cultures from peripheral blood were positive for *Abiotrophia defectiva* bacteremia, which was attributed to recent MWA since the patient had fevers/chills after the ablation. Patient required hospitalization for 8 days and was treated with combination of 4 vancomycin and 14-day course of ceftriaxone.

Complication Analysis

Percutaneous drainage could be considered the optimal management in this case. Aspiration alone was attempted initially as the collection was too small for drainage placement with the hope that this could resolve and be completely treated with antibiotics. The patient improved on antimicrobial therapy and additional intervention was not performed, although the patient was a high-risk patient for biliary complications due to pre-existing large biloma, baseline biliary dilatation, and history of bevacizumab and HAIP chemotherapy exposure.

Approximately 1 month later, patient presented with abdominal pain, fever, and leucocytosis. Repeat contrast-enhanced CT scan demonstrated communicating bilomas with secondary biliary duct compression: A new segment 3 biloma (10.3 × 8.3 cm in size) at the site of the MWA zone was now seen in addition to the postsurgical segment 4 biloma (11.2 × 8.6 cm in size), present before the MWA (▶ Fig. 3.120). Patient underwent endoscopic retrograde cholangiopancreatography

(ERCP) and stenting with metal stent due to biliary duct compression, secondary to the postresection segment 4 biloma. Additionally, the patient underwent CT, ultrasound, and fluoroscopy-guided drainage of communicating bilomas from anterolateral position (▶ Fig. 3.121). A total of 650 mL of biliary fluid was drained, completely evacuating the collection; microbiology cultures were negative. Patient received premedication of cefotan and fentanyl.

Nine days postbiloma drainage, patient developed high biloma drain output (> 1 L/day). The patient underwent ERCP, which showed malignantly-appearing biliary stricture and biliary leak into the biloma at the resection site. Bare metal stent was placed into a common bile duct for the biliary stricture management. Upon identification of connection between the new biloma and the left biliary tree, pericatheter biliary leakage around biloma drain was managed: the biloma catheter was exchanged for a 6 French brite tip sheath (Cordis, Milpitas, CA, USA). Using a Bernstein catheter (Angiodynamics, Latham, NY, USA) and hydrophilic GLIDEWIRE (Terumo, Tokyo, Japan) the left biliary tree was accessed from the biloma cavity and the wire was positioned into the duodenum. The hydrophilic wire was exchanged for a stiff *Amplatz* (Boston Scientific, Marlborough, MA, USA). An internal–external biliary catheter was placed for diversion of bile to allow healing of the biliary leak.

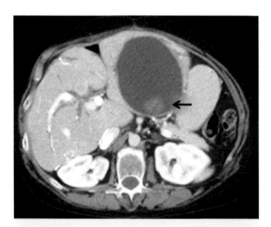

Fig. 3.120 Follow-up contrast-enhanced CT scan again obtained when patient was symptomatic. A large fluid collection was identified. A small amount of higher attenuating material was seen layering likely representing small amount of debris or hemorrhage (*arrow*). This collection was drained percutaneously.

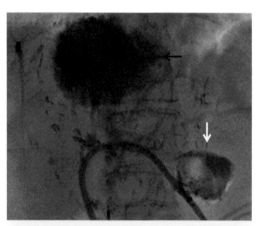

Fig. 3.121 Placement of a biliary drain for appropriate diversion and expedited healing. The biliary tree was accessed from the biloma with placement of an internal–external biliary drain for biliary diversion. Cholangiogram demonstrated a connection between the preablation surgical biloma in segment 4 (*black arrow*) and the new segment 2/3 biloma (*white arrow*).

Drainage of postablation segment 3 biloma continued on last follow-up, with biloma size of 3.4 × 3.1 cm. There was a plan to drain postsurgical segment 4 biloma 9.6 × 7.1 cm in size and then rebuild biliary tree with stents on last follow-up.

The patient had no local tumor progression on last follow-up in ablation zone, with Local-tumor-progression-free-survival (LTPFS) of 10.7 months. Patient was alive on last follow-up 1 year post-procedure.

Strategies to Prevent and Take-Home Message

- When treating secondary liver malignancies with a curative intent using percutaneous thermal ablation, minimal ablation margins greater than 5 mm and ideally 10 mm circumferentially are necessary to achieve long term local tumor control.
- Be aware of increased risk of biliary complications in patients with history of HAIP therapy and pre-existing liver biliary problems (biloma, bile duct dilatation).

- In patients with above mentioned biliary complications risk factors, consider less aggressive ablation, creating 5 to 10 mm minimal ablation margin, but not exceeding 10 mm.
- In postablation, when patient is symptomatic, especially in the presence of fever and leukocytosis, a gas and fluid containing liver collection should be considered as an abscess until proven otherwise. Treatment should include the administration of a broad spectrum intravenous antibiotic and urgent drainage of the collection.

Further Reading

Kurilova I, Boas EKF, Yarmohammadi H, et al. Review of complications following thermal ablation of colorerctal cancer liver metastases. J Vasc Interv Radiol. 2018

Ito K, Ito H, Kemeny NE, et al. Biliary sclerosis after hepatic arterial infusion pump chemotherapy for patients with colorectal cancer liver metastasis: incidence, clinical features, and risk factors. Ann Surg Oncol. 2012; 19(5):1609–1617

Cercek A, D'Angelica M, Power D, et al. Floxuridine hepatic arterial infusion associated biliary toxicity is increased by concurrent administration of systemic bevacizumab. Ann Surg Oncol. 2014; 21(2):479–486

3.5.7 Hip Joint Destruction following Radiofrequency Ablation and Cementoplasty of an Adjacent Bone Metastasis

Patient History

A 50-year-old woman suffered from a breast cancer. She developed a single and asymptomatic bone metastasis localized in the left acetabulum (▶ Fig. 3.122). The metastasis is slowly progressive and a local curative treatment was decided at tumor board. Radiofrequency ablation (RFA) was the chosen option in order to obtain a biopsy during the same procedure, but also to perform a prophylactic consolidation using cementoplasty.

Initial Treatment and Imaging Plan

Technically, the procedure was performed under general anesthesia and CT-guidance. Two bone-access needles were used to enter the upper and the lower part of the metastasis. A biopsy was performed and subsequently confirmed the diagnostic of breast metastasis. Then, an RFA probe (2 cm active tip, Cooltip, Covidien; Medtronic, Minneapolis,

MN, USA) was inserted through each bone-access needles (▶ Fig. 3.123) in order to perform two successive thermal ablations (5 minutes each, resulting in a final temperature around 80 °C at the tip of the probe at the end of the procedure). Finally, polymethylmethacrylate cement was injected into the bone metastasis using both access needles (▶ Fig. 3.124). This 1-hour procedure was considered successful and the patient discharged the day after.

Problems Encountered during the Treatment

None.

Resulting Complication

At 1-month follow-up, the patient complained of severe hip pain, which appeared within few days after the procedure. The MRI demonstrated a

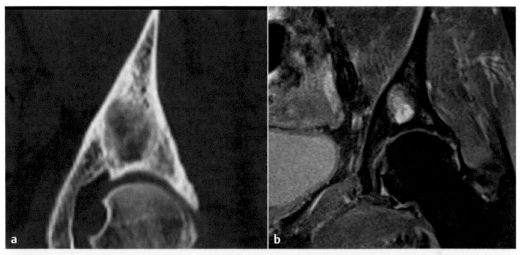

Fig. 3.122 Single bone metastasis located in the acetabulum. CT scan is shown in (a) and MRI is shown in (b).

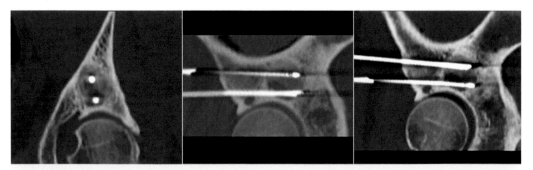

Fig. 3.123 Multiplanar CT reconstruction images showing the insertion of two bone access needles to perform two successive thermal ablations at the upper and the lower part of the metastasis.

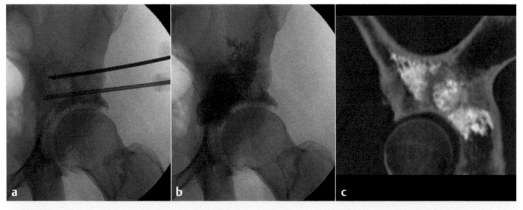

Fig. 3.124 Cementoplasty for prophylactic consolidation during fluroscopy (a,b) and CT reconstruction (c).

complete destruction of the bone metastasis with nice safety margins but also an important inflammatory process in the area of the ablated zone (▶ Fig. 3.125).

Steroids improved the pain during the following weeks but thereafter slowly increased over time. One year after the procedure the patient was unable to walk more than 100 m. X-ray of the hip demonstrated a rapid degenerative process of the coxofemoral joint requiring a total hip arthroplasty (▶ Fig. 3.126).

Complication Analysis and Complication Management

The main reason for this degenerative process is related to thermal damage to the join with: (1) bone necrosis of the femoral head, and (2) deterioration of both the femoral head and the acetabular aspects of the hip joint. The patient required a total hip arthroplasty at 1 year after treatment.

Strategies to Prevent and Take-Home Message

- Be aware of the potential threat of thermal ablation near joint surfaces due to damage to adjacent articular cartilage.
- Consider arthroscopy assisted RFA with fluid irrigation during the procedure.

Further Reading

Issack PS, Kotwal SY, Lane JM. Management of metastatic bone disease of the acetabulum. J Am Acad Orthop Surg. 2013; 21 (11):685–695

Lane MD, Le HB, Lee S, et al. Combination radiofrequency ablation and cementoplasty for palliative treatment of painful neoplastic bone metastasis: experience with 53 treated lesions in 36 patients. Skeletal Radiol. 2011; 40(1):25–32

Jakanani GC, Jaiveer S, Ashford R, Rennie W. Computed tomography-guided coblation and cementoplasty of a painful acetabular metastasis: an effective palliative treatment. J Palliat Med. 2010; 13(1):83–85

Zoric BB, Horn N, Braun S, Millett PJ. Factors influencing intra-articular fluid temperature profiles with radiofrequency ablation. J Bone Joint Surg Am. 2009; 91(10):2448–2454

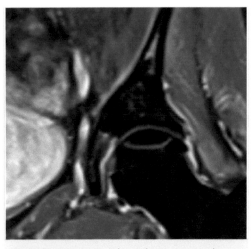

Fig. 3.125 T1 contrast enhanced MRI at 1 month demonstrated a complete destruction of the bone metastasis.

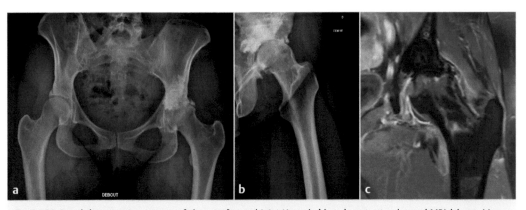

Fig. 3.126 Rapid degenerative process of the coxofemoral joint X-ray **(a,b)** and contrast enhanced MRI **(c)** requiring a total hip arthroplasty at 1 year.

3.5.8 Calyceal Leakage after Renal Biopsy

Patient History

In a 52-year-old female patient, a 1.8 cm exophytic lesion with calcifications was discovered as an incidental finding during an abdominal ultrasound evaluation for upper abdominal quadrants. Although patient was explained the active surveillance option, she chose to go for biopsy upon agreement of the urologist in charge.

Initial Treatment Received

Under local anesthesia, strict sterility measures and CT-guided percutaneous biopsy was performed using an 18-gauge semiautomatic soft-tissue biopsy needle (▶ Fig. 3.127).

Problems Encountered during the Treatment

About 4 hours later the patient reported severe pain and vomiting.

Imaging Plan

A new CT scan without contrast injection was performed, which showed a large amount of contrast medium around the kidney, most probably from calyceal leakage.

Resulting Complication

The new CT scan without contrast injection showed a large amount of contrast medium around the kidney, most probably from calyceal leakage (▶ Fig. 3.128).

Possible Strategies for Complication Management

- Intravenous antibiosis.
- Percutaneous drainage.
- Percutaneous nephrostomy.
- Surgical operation.

What Would You Do?

Notes:

_____

_____

_____

_____

_____

_____

_____

_____

Final Complication Management

A nephrostomy was percutaneously placed under fluoroscopy and ultrasound guidance. Patient was hospitalized for 2 days; intravenous antibiosis was administrated. Resolution of symptoms post 2 days (▶ Fig. 3.129).

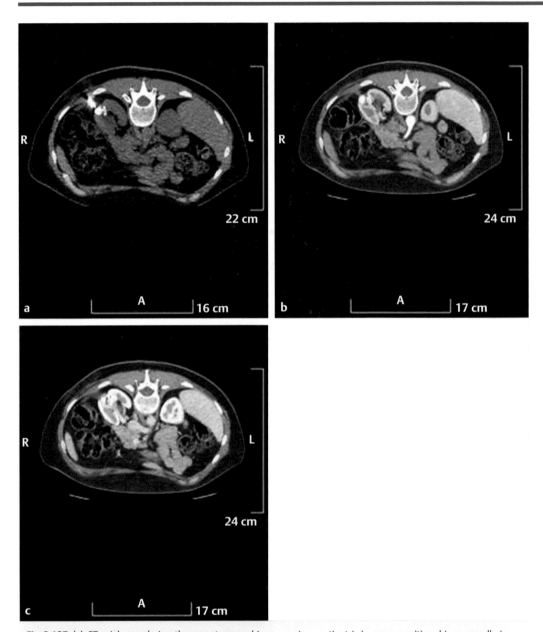

Fig. 3.127 **(a)** CT axial scan during the percutaneous biopsy session—patient is in prone position; biopsy needle is located right next to the lesion. **(b, c)** Immediate post biopsy CT axial scan postcontrast medium injection in arterial **(b)** and venous **(c)** phases revealed no sign of extravasation.

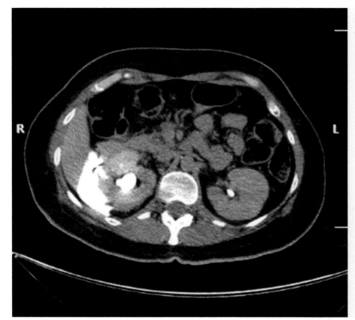

Fig. 3.128 CT axial scan 4 hours after the biopsy session—a large amount of contrast medium around the kidney most probably from calyceal leakage.

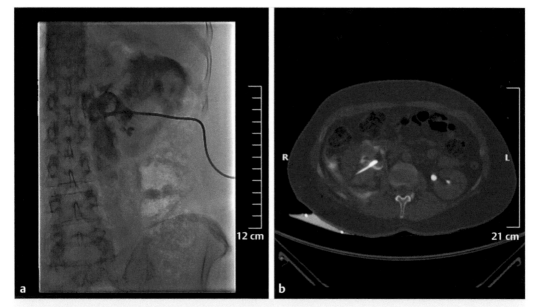

Fig. 3.129 **(a)** Fluoroscopy posteroanterior view: nephrostomy catheter is in position. **(b)** CT axial scans immediately after nephrostomy placement—the catheter is placed in the renal pelvis through the calyceal system of the lower kidney; there is still contrast medium in the perinephric space.

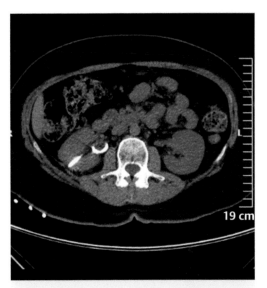

Fig. 3.130 CT axial scan 1 month postoperative. A new CT scan was performed 4 hours post intravenous contrast medium injection; there were no fluids or contrast medium leakage. Nephrostomy catheter was removed.

Complication Analysis

There was no real lesion; instead the biopsy target was a renal milk of calcium cyst found within a calyceal diverticulum (▶ Fig. 3.130).

Strategies to Prevent and Take-Home Message

- Renal milk of calcium cysts is a term referring to calcium precipitate located either within a calyceal diverticulum that has lost communication with the collecting system, or within a simple renal cyst.
- Hemorrhage requiring overnight hospital admission in 2% of the cases.
- Pre-procedural evaluation of imaging is of utmost importance.

Further Reading

Catalano OA, Samir AE. Renal biopsy. In: Interventional Radiology Procedures in Biopsy and Drainage. Gervais DA, Sabharwal T, eds. Lee M, Watkinson A, Series eds. London: Springer; 59–65

Khan SA, Khan FR, Fletcher MS, Richenberg JL. Milk of calcium (MOC) cysts masquerading as renal calculi—a trap for the unwary. Cent European J Urol. 2012; 65(3):170–173

Huang YS, Huang KH, Chang CC, Liu KL. Milk of calcium in abdomen. Urology. 2011; 77(3):596–597

3.5.9 Hemopericardium Following Malplacement of a Radiofrequency Ablation Electrode during Thermal Ablation of the Liver—A Potentially Fatal Complication

Patient History

A 50-year-old male patient with colorectal cancer presented to our department following surgical resection of the primary tumor and atypical resection of synchronous liver mets. Two of the liver mets had not be resected, one centrally in the right liver lobe, the other located in segment II/III. Tumor board consensus was to perform thermal ablation on both of the remaining lesions (▶ Fig. 3.131).

Initial Treatment and Imaging Plan

The procedure was performed under general anesthesia using CT-image guidance. During the first part of the procedure, a metastasis in the central right lobe was successfully ablated without complications. Needle placement was performed during periods of breath-hold with monitoring of ablation using incremental CT images.

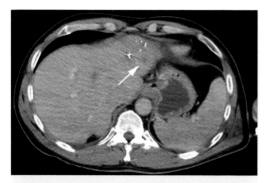

Fig. 3.131 Axial contrast-enhanced CT of a 1.5 cm metastasis in the left liver lobe (*arrow*).

Problems Encountered during Treatment

The metastasis in segment II/III was successfully targeted with a 22-gauge Chiba puncture needle, which was placed to guide tracking of the radiofrequency electrode. Due to the previous surgery with atypical resection of a subcapsular lesion in segment II, the target lesion was surrounded by hard scar tissue impeding penetration of the electrode. During insertion of the 14-gauge radiofrequency ablation (RFA) needle (12 cm Talon Semiflex, Angiodynamics; Queensbury, NY, USA), the device took an unplanned course and followed the capsule of the left lobe cranially into the direction of the heart. Initial control CT after needle advancement showed position of the needle tip close to the base of the right ventricle, possibly within the peri- and/or myocardium (▶ Fig. 3.132).

Resulting Complication

Malpositioning of the RFA electrode within or near the heart with possible penetration. To further determine the exact position of the device, a contrast-enhanced CT scan was performed. Multiplanar reconstruction showed that the needle tip was lying directly adjacent to the base of the right ventricle. There were no signs of active bleeding (▶ Fig. 3.133, ▶ Fig. 3.134).

Complication Analysis and Complication Management

Advancement of the 14-gauge needle was not performed under CT fluoroscopy or real-time ultrasound guidance. Incremental CT slices were used for planning and navigation only.

Despite a slight resistance felt during needle insertion, the electrode was advanced "blindly."

Once the malpositioning had been detected, echocardiography was performed, which revealed that the electrode had not penetrated the myocardium, but was, in fact, located in the pericardial sac. Under ultrasound guidance, the device was removed and a three-phased contrast enhanced control CT was performed. There were no signs of active bleeding. However, a 2 cm hemopericardium developed, reaching the pericardial fold at the aortic root.

During the initial procedure and after device removal, the patient remained hemodynamically stable. He was kept intubated and echocardiographic controls were performed every half hour. About 2 hours following the procedure, there was no progression of hemopericardium and the patient was extubated. He was without any symptoms and recovered uneventfully. During the follow-up, the pericardial effusion resolved completely. The patient was referred to the surgical department for surgical resection of the remaining metastasis of the left liver lobe.

Strategies to Prevent and Take-Home Message

- Beware of the potential threat of thermal ablation electrodes near the adjacent organs. Puncturing vital organs is potentially fatal.
- For procedure planning, topography of anatomic structures must be assessed in multiple plains.
- CT fluoroscopy or real-time ultrasound should be used to assist RFA needle placement.
- Consider fluid irrigation (artificial pleural effusion or artificial ascites) as water-lock for targeting difficult lesions.
- Pericardial tamponade is a rare but serious complication of liver ablation and might be due to thermal damage or direct puncture.

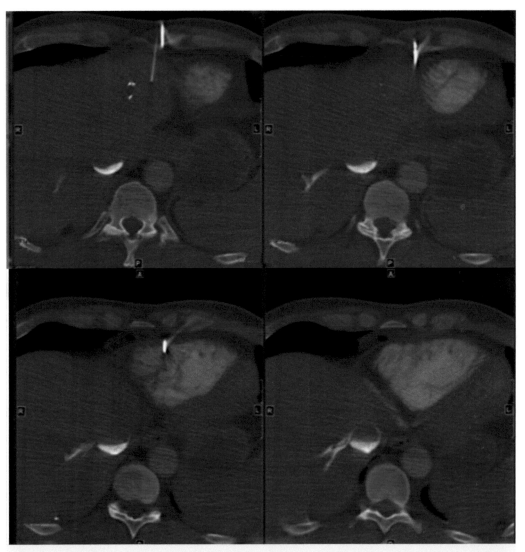

Fig. 3.132 Initial axial control CT revealing pericardial position of the tip of the electrode outside the liver. The 22-gauge needle still in place near the metastasis.

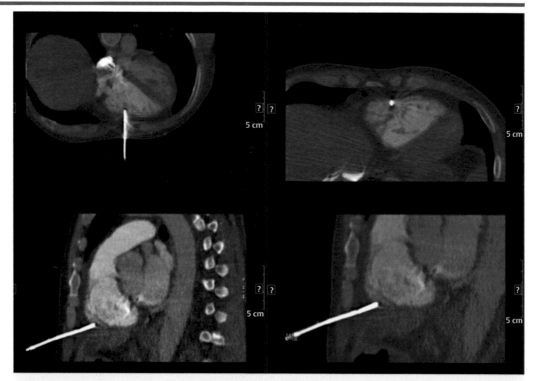

Fig. 3.133 Multiplanar contrast enhanced CT imaging of the malplaced radiofrequency ablation electrode excluding active bleeding from the punctured heart.

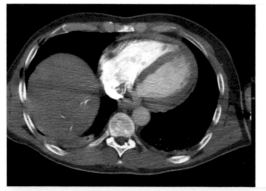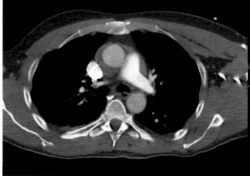

Fig. 3.134 Contrast enhanced axial CT showing pericardial effusion consistent with hemopericardium.

Further Reading

Chung MW, Ha SY, Choi JH, et al. Cardiac tamponade after radiofrequency ablation for hepatocellular carcinoma: case report and literature review. Medicine (Baltimore). 2018; 97(49):e13532

Kwon HJ, Kim PN, Byun JH, et al. Various complications of percutaneous radiofrequency ablation for hepatic tumors: radiologic findings and technical tips. Acta Radiol. 2014; 55(9):1082–1092

Rhim H, Yoon KH, Lee JM, et al. Major complications after radiofrequency thermal ablation of hepatic tumors: spectrum of imaging findings. Radiographics. 2003; 23(1):123–134, discussion 134–136

Loh KB, Bux SI, Abdullah BJ, Raja Mokhtar RA, Mohamed R. Hemorrhagic cardiac tamponade: rare complication of radiofrequency ablation of hepatocellular carcinoma. Korean J Radiol. 2012; 13(5):643–647

Gao J, Sun WB, Tong ZC, Ding XM, Ke S. Successful treatment of acute hemorrhagic cardiac tamponade in a patient with hepatocellular carcinoma during percutaneous radiofrequency ablation. Chin Med J (Engl). 2010; 123(11):1470–1472

Silverman ER, Lai YH, Osborn IP, Yudkowitz FS. Percutaneous radiofrequency ablation of hepatocellular lesions in segment II of the liver: a risk factor for cardiac tamponade. J Clin Anesth. 2013; 25(7):587–590

3.5.10 Infection of the Ablation Cave after Electrochemotherapy of a Colorectal Liver Metastasis

Patient History

A 70-year-old female patient presented with a rapidly progredient solitary liver metastasis of the underlying cecal rectal cancer. Primary origin was confirmed by biopsy. Due to preceded surgical hemihepatectomy, the reserve of the remnant liver was considerably restricted. After rectal surgery, chemoradiation, and hemihepatectomy, the only site of persistent and progressive malignancy was the target lesion in the remnant liver. This solitary liver metastasis, consistent with a recurrent metastasis at the resection edge was progredient under different systemic chemotherapies, at least including the full range of available drugs 5-fluorouracil/leucovorin combined with oxaliplatin (FOLFOX) and irinotecan (FOLFIRI), capecitabine, bevacizumab, and trifluridine/tipiracil. A starting cholestasis was treated with a biliary stent. Because of the size (10 cm diameter) and localization, there were no therapeutic options for repeated surgery, as well as for thermal ablation including radiofrequency, microwave, and cryoablation (Fig. 3.135). The decision for a stereotactic radiation therapy has to be eliminated due to the large dimension of the target lesion. The interdisciplinary decision

voted for the local therapy using electroconvulsive therapy (ECT). The main reason was to avoid expected secondary complications. Despite of the multiple prior therapies, the patient had an unimpaired performance status (Karnofsky 90%/ECOG 0).

Initial Treatment Received

CT-guided electrochemotherapy of the liver (Fig. 3.136, Fig. 3.137, Fig. 3.138).

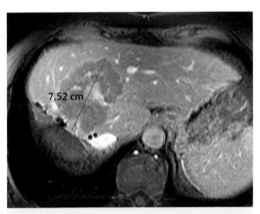

Fig. 3.135 Contrast enhanced MRI of the target lesion in the remnant liver, supposedly a recurrent metastasis at the resection edge after hemihepatectomy.

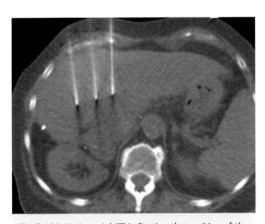

Fig. 3.136 Native axial CT indicating the position of the electroconvulsive therapy applicators. Previously 15 mg of bleomycin was administered intravenously. Approximately 8 minutes after intravenous administration of bleomycin the electroporation occurred.

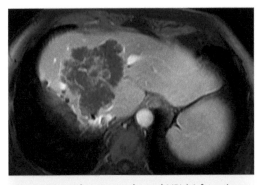

Fig. 3.137 Axial contrast enhanced MRI (t1 fat sat) showing the ablation hole 2 days after electroconvulsive therapy. A sufficient chemoablation of the entire target lesion can be demonstrated.

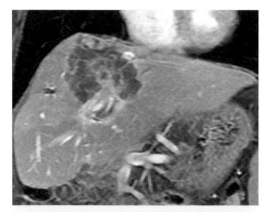

Fig. 3.138 Electroconvulsive therapy has the ability to preserve vascular structures. Imaging characteristics for an abscess formation were not detectable at any time point of follow-up imaging (Contrast enhanced MRI).

Problems Encountered during the Treatment

Increased inflammatory parameters after ECT, those persisted for 3 weeks. Otherwise a technically successful chemoablation, and altogether an unremarkable procedure. No further complications were reported.

Imaging Plan

Contrast-enhanced MRI of the liver.

Resulting Complication

Subclinical infection of the ablation hole, supposedly via the enclosed biliary stent.

Possible Strategies for Complication Management

- Oral, better intravenous administration of targeted antibiotic therapy.
- Abscess drainage, if required.
- Surgery (if abscess drainage fails).

Final Complication Management

Intravenous antibiotic therapy (ciprofloxacin and metronidazole).

Complication Analysis

ECT of a large liver malignancy and indwelling biliary stent resulted in a local infection.

Strategies to Prevent and Take-Home Message

- Already pre-interventional prophylactic antibiotic therapy at least 5 days before intervention.
- Fasting for 2 to 3 days before intervention to reduce the intestinal flora.

Further Reading

Tarantino L, Busto G, Nasto A, et al. Electrochemotherapy of cholangiocellular carcinoma at hepatic hilum: a feasibility study. Eur J Surg Oncol. 2018; 44(10):1603–1609

Campana LG, Edhemovic I, Soden D, et al. Electrochemotherapy—emerging applications technical advances, new indications, combined approaches, and multi-institutional collaboration. Eur J Surg Oncol. 2019; 45(2):92–102

Cornelis FH, Korenbaum C, Ben Ammar M, Tavolaro S, Nouri-Neuville M, Lotz JP. Multimodal image-guided electrochemotherapy of unresectable liver metastasis from renal cell cancer. Diagn Interv Imaging. 2019:2211–5684

3.6 Vascular Miscellaneous Cases

3.6.1 Arterioportal Fistula Following Microwave Ablation of Subcentimeter Liver Metastasis from Sigmoid Adenocarcinoma

Patient History

A 68-year-old female was diagnosed with sigmoid adenocarcinoma 4 years prior. She received systemic chemotherapy and underwent a laparoscopic left hemicolectomy. On routine follow-up cross-sectional imaging approximately 2 years later, she was found to have new hepatic metastases, which

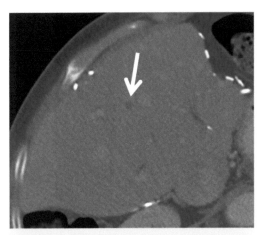

Fig. 3.139 Contrast-enhanced CT scan with a new 7 mm hypoattenuating hepatic tumor adjacent to a branch of the right portal vein (*arrow*).

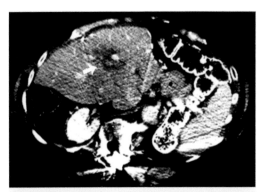

Fig. 3.140 Intra-procedural CT scan demonstrating extended ablation zone (*arrow*).

were treated with resection and direct intra-arterial chemotherapy via the placement of a hepatic artery infusion pump. After approximately 1 year, patient was found to have a 7 × 7 mm hypodense tumor near the portal vein, consistent with progression of disease within the liver (▶ Fig. 3.139). After multidisciplinary discussion, she was deemed a good candidate for percutaneous microwave ablation (MWA).

Initial Treatment

Percutaneous MWA of a subcentimeter recurrent colon cancer hepatic metastasis was performed. Ultrasound, CT, and a split dose ^{18}F-FDG PET/CT technique were used for tumor localization and MWA probe placement. Split dose ^{18}F-FDG PET/CT technique and contrast-enhanced CT were used for evaluation of ablation technical success.

Given the subcentimeter size of the tumor, a single Neuwave ablation PR15 electrode (Ethicon, Madison, WI, USA) was utilized. Total of four overlapping "low and slow" ablations, utilizing relatively depressed power of 35 W for 10 minutes were performed to avoid damage to the adjacent portal vein. Two overlaps were performed for initial ablation, however, due to inadequate inferior ablation margin demonstrated on contrast-enhanced CT; the lesion was reablated with two additional overlaps. Minimal ablation margin of 5 mm from hepatic vein was achieved, with 8 mm at inferior margin and more than 10 mm around the rest of tumor, with ablation zone measurements of 2.8 × 2.5 × 2.4 cm.

A triple-phase CT and split dose ^{18}F-FDG PET/CT were performed at the end of the second ablation cycle (▶ Fig. 3.140). No metabolic uptake and no contrast enhancement within the ablation zone were noted. A hypodense area measuring approximately 28 × 24 × 25 mm was identified corresponding to the immediate posttreatment ablation zone. Patient was asymptomatic and further was planned to be managed with expectant observation.

Problems Encountered during the Treatment

None. Patient was successfully treated with MWA. Both immediate postablation ^{18}F-FDG PET/CT and three-phase contrast-enhanced CT scan demonstrated complete ablation of the tumor. No vascular abnormalities were noted.

Imaging Plan

Patient was scheduled for routine postablation multiphase CT scan 1 month postablation, which served as a new baseline imaging for future comparisons.

Resulting Complication

On follow-up imaging at 3.5 months post-MWA, geographic hyperperfusion ablation area was incidentally noted on an arterial phase imaging. In the region of the ablation defect, distal portal venous branches displayed similar attenuation to adjacent hepatic arteries on the arterial phase, when proximal portal vein showed normal expected attenuation. These findings were suggestive of an intrahepatic arterioportal shunt (▶ Fig. 3.141).

What Would You Do?

Notes:

_____

_____

_____

_____

_____

_____

_____

_____

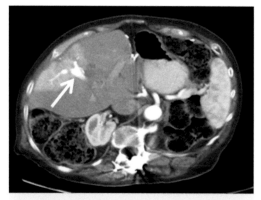

Fig. 3.141 Arterial phase CT perfusion abnormalities surrounding the ablation zone. Distal portal venous hyperattenuation (*arrow*) similar to hepatic arterial branches, proximal portal vein shows normal expected attenuation.

no further visualization of the portal vein was achieved (▶ Fig. 3.142a, b).

Patient did not develop local tumor progression with local tumor progression-free survival of 36.6 months; however, patient developed disease progression in untreated liver. Patient was alive on last follow-up 5 years postablation.

Possible Strategies for Complication Management

- Embolization of the arterioportal shunt.
- Conservative "watch and wait" with close imaging follow-up is not recommended as it has a long-term risk of portal hypertension and liver failure.

Final Complication Management

A diagnostic arteriogram was performed. Digital subtraction angiography (DSA) was performed in the superior mesenteric, celiac, and right hepatic arteries. A PROGREAT microcatheter (Terumo, Sumerset, NJ, USA) was advanced into the right hepatic artery. DSA demonstrated distal hepatic artery communication to the distal portal vein branch with rapid arterioportal flow. Embolization was performed utilizing detachable Ruby coils (Penumbra, Alameda, CA, USA) and Gelfoam Sterile Compressed Sponge (Pfizer, New York City, NY, USA) until occlusion of arterioportal fistula with

Complication Analysis

Damage to adjacent structures such as hepatic arteries, hepatic and portal veins, or bile ducts are well known, although rare complications following thermal ablation. When treating secondary liver malignancies with a curative intent using percutaneous ablation, minimal ablation margins greater than 5 mm and ideally 10 mm circumferentially are necessary to achieve long-term local tumor control. However, this minimal ablation margin cannot always be achieved, especially when lesions are centrally located and adjacent to large central vessels that impact the deposition of heat in the tumor through the heat sink phenomenon. MWA has been shown to be less influenced by this than MWA. In this case, we presented the MWA of the lesion, located in a very close proximity to a portal vein branch. This impacted the ability to create adequate minimal ablation margin and required additional ablation to extend the ablation zone into the pulmonary vein branch with subsequent development of portal injury and arterioportal

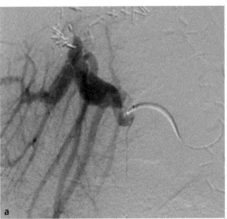 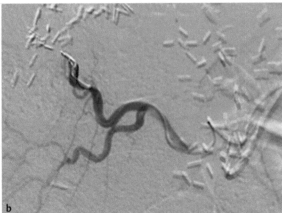

Fig. 3.142 (a) Selective digital subtraction angiography of the right hepatic artery demonstrated filling of the adjacent portal vein with hepatofugal flow of contrast. **(b)** Postembolization imaging.

shunt. The patient was completely asymptomatic, thus a conservative "watch and wait" approach could have been undertaken although this could cause portal hypertension and eventual liver failure. Therefore, a decision to repair the fistula was obtained.

Small hepatic arterioportal shunts usually have limited clinical significance. However, in a percentage of patients over time, if untreated, these abnormalities could cause significant abnormal hepatic perfusion and portal hypertension. These shunts are of increased importance when considering transcatheter arterial therapy. In case transcatheter arterial therapy is considered, embolization should be attempted prior to treating the tumor, given the large size and brisk flow of the shunt.

Strategies to Prevent and Take-Home Message

- When treating secondary liver malignancies with a curative intent using percutaneous ablation, minimal ablation margins greater than 5 mm and ideally 10 mm circumferentially are necessary to achieve long-term local tumor control.
- In case the lesion is in close proximity to major hepatic structures and adequate ablation margin cannot be safely achieved and the lesion is relatively small (< 1 cm), consider using alternative nonthermal ablation modality, such as irreversible electroporation, which enables to spare blood vessels and bile ducts.
- When using MWA for the lesions in close proximity to the blood vessels and bile ducts, utilize relatively depressed ablation power for "low and slow" ablations.
- Small hepatic arterioportal shunts usually have limited clinical significance. However, in the long run, if untreated, these abnormalities could potentially cause significant abnormal hepatic perfusion and portal hypertension. These shunts are of increased importance when considering transcatheter arterial therapy and embolization should be attempted prior to treating the tumor in case of large size and brisk flow of the shunt.

Further Reading

Lahat E, Eshkenazy R, Zendel A, et al. Complications after percutaneous ablation of liver tumors: a systematic review. Hepatobiliary Surg Nutr. 2014; 3(5):317–323

Ding J, Jing X, Liu J, et al. Complications of thermal ablation of hepatic tumours: comparison of radiofrequency and microwave ablative techniques. Clin Radiol. 2013; 68(6):608–615

Bertot LC, Sato M, Tateishi R, Yoshida H, Koike K. Mortality and complication rates of percutaneous ablative techniques for the treatment of liver tumors: a systematic review. Eur Radiol. 2011; 21(12):2584–2596

3.6.2 Arteriovenous Fistula after Diagnostic Renal Puncture

Patient History

A 73-year-old male patient with a chronic renal failure was scheduled for a renal biopsy of the right kidney in order to diagnose the underlying unknown renal disease. Patient's medical history and laboratory values were reviewed, with particular attention to coagulation profile and creatinine level, which appeared normal.

Initial Treatment

Imaging-guided percutaneous biopsy of the lower pole was performed with conscious sedation under ultrasound guidance (▶ Fig. 3.143). The lower pole is commonly selected with a posterior approach, in order to follow the avascular line of Brodie, minimizing complications.

Problems Encountered during the Treatment

Two hours after the biopsy, the patient showed acute macrohaematuria with lowering laboratoristic data associated with right flank pain.

Imaging Plan

A transfemoral renal artery angiography was performed. It demonstrated an anomalous renal arteriovenous fistula at the lower pole of the kidney (▶ Fig. 3.144), causing shunting of arterialized blood into the low-pressure venous system.

What Would You Do?

Notes:

_____

_____

_____

_____

_____

_____

_____

_____

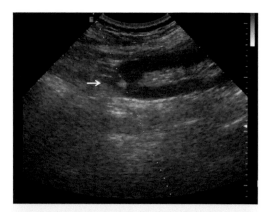

Fig. 3.143 Longitudinal sonogram of right kidney shows the hyperechoic tip of an 18-gauges needle sampling a portion of parenchyma at the lower pole (*arrow*).

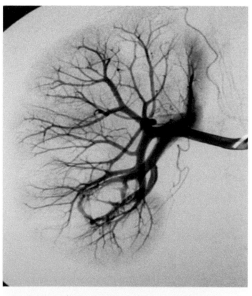

Fig. 3.144 Selective right renal artery angiogram demonstrates the arteriovenous fistula with early opacification of the draining vein at the lower pole.

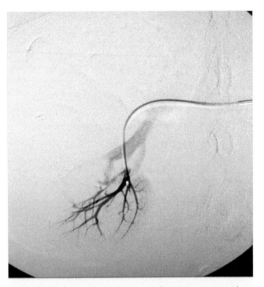

Fig. 3.145 Superselective lower pole arteriogram with the microcatheter in the feeding artery.

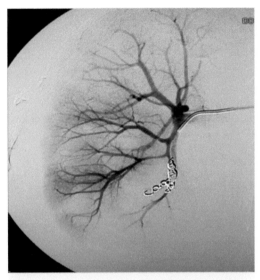

Fig. 3.146 Selective renal postembolization angiogram demonstrates several microcoils at the site of fistula. Neither a fistula, nor early venous filling is observed.

Possible Strategies for Complication Management

- Transarterial selective angioembolization.
- Surgery (partial or total nephrectomy).
- Combination of transarterial selective angioembolization and surgery.

Final Complication Management

A selective transarterial coil embolization was performed. A right common femoral artery was catheterized until the site of arteriovenous fistula (▶ Fig. 3.145) and several microcoils were deployed in the feeding vessel (▶ Fig. 3.146).

Complication Analysis

During the biopsy, a needle passed through both an artery and a vein, determining this anomalous communication. Even if this is a potentially life-threatening condition, if quickly recognized it can be treated by interventional radiology. Angiography not only demonstrates the anatomic location of fistula, but it also allows the intervention. Prior angiography, a contrast-enhanced CT might help to identify the source of bleeding for further planning of the interventional procedure and it gives an impression of further changes intra-abdominal resulting from a potential bleeding complication.

Strategies to Prevent and Take-Home Message

- It is very important before a renal biopsy to evaluate the coagulation profile.
- A careful post-biopsy period of observation is necessary.
- Embolization is a useful technique for treatment of renal arteriovenous fistula.

Further Reading

Sosa-Barrios RH, Burguera V, Rodriguez-Mendiola N, et al. Arteriovenous fistulae after renal biopsy: diagnosis and outcomes using Doppler ultrasound assessment. BMC Nephrol. 2017; 18(1):365

Feldmann Y, Böer K, Wolf G, Busch M. Complications and monitoring of percutaneous renal biopsy—a retrospective study. Clin Nephrol. 2018; 89(4):260–268

Maruno M, Kiyosue H, Tanoue S, et al. Renal arteriovenous shunts: clinical features, imaging appearance, and transcatheter embolization based on angioarchitecture. Radiographics. 2016; 36(2): 580–595

3.6.3 Laceration of the Left Hepatic Artery during Biliary Drainage

Patient History

A 70 year-old-male with negative previous history was presented with obstructive jaundice and cholangitis. The initial ultrasound examination revealed presence of bile duct dilatation and solid liver lesions. A CT followed and confirmed the presence of a solid mass of the head of pancreas that was causing biliary obstruction and the presence of multiple liver metastases; the staging of the lesion was T2 N0 M1. Biliary drainage was recommended followed by biopsy of one of the liver lesions.

Initial Treatment

Endoscopic retrograde cholangiopancreatography failed and percutaneous drainage was decided. Written informed consent was obtained. Ultrasound-guided puncture of the left liver lobe under aseptic technique, local anesthesia, and conscious sedation followed. A cholangiogram confirmed the level of occlusion at the distal common bile duct and an 8.5 French catheter was inserted. The liver lesion was biopsied and confirmed metastatic nature and the patient was considered for palliative treatment. Internalization of the drain with a metallic stent was decided. The procedure was performed under general anesthesia. The distal common bile duct lesion was crossed with a hydrophilic wire and an 8 mm × 10 cm self-expanding biliary stent was deployed. Brushing samples from the lesion were obtained for cytology. An 8.5 French internal–external biliary drain was left in situ.

Problems Encountered during the Treatment

Significant bleeding was detected when the internal–external drain was inserted. Regular flush of the drain was recommended. Suggestion to remove the drain a week later was made. The cholangiogram revealed no significant dilatation in the biliary tree but almost complete blockage of the biliary stent from blood clots (▶ Fig. 3.147). A new general anesthesia procedure was organized, as

patient could not tolerate procedure under sedation. The biliary drain has been removed over a wire and a 6 French sheath has been inserted. The cholangiogram revealed presence of filling defects at the distal end of the stent. Cleaning of the stent with a balloon was attempted but was not effective. A new endoscopically removable 10 mm × 10 cm covered stent was deployed inside the previous one (▶ Fig. 3.148). The final cholangiographic result was satisfactory, moderate bleeding occurred during the procedure and an 8.5 French internal–external drain was left in situ. Drain removal was arranged for 4 days later under local anesthesia and mild sedation. While the drain was removed over a wire, brisk, pulsatile blood returned from the puncture site and the patient became immediately hypotensive and tachycardia. A new 10 French drain was inserted over the wire and fluid resuscitation followed.

Imaging Plan

A CT angiogram has been immediately been performed and did not show any area of contrast

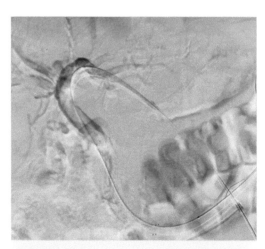

Fig. 3.147 Cholangiogram a week after initial stent insertion that reveals nearly complete blockage of the biliary stent from clot and no contrast in the duodenum.

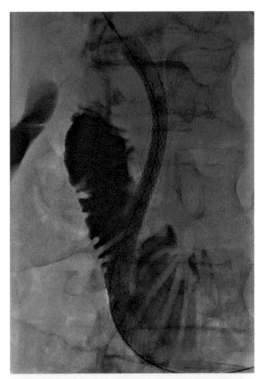

Fig. 3.148 A 10 mm × 10 cm covered stent was inserted into the previous stent after cleaning the clot with a balloon. Satisfactory contrast drain toward the bowel.

extravasation. The close vicinity of the drain to a small left hepatic artery branch was noted.

Resulting Complication

Laceration of the left hepatic artery during biliary drainage procedure.

Possible Strategies for Complication Management

- Keep the biliary drain in situ.
- Perform immediate angiogram in view of embolization.
- Consider surgical options.
- Upsize the biliary drain.

Final Complication Management

Immediate embolization of the left hepatic artery branch was decided. Procedure was performed under local anesthesia. Access was obtained from the right common femoral artery. Retrograde puncture, 6 French sheath. Selective catheterization of the common hepatic artery. Angiogram did not confirm any contrast extravasation when the biliary drain was in situ (▶ Fig. 3.149). When the biliary drain was carefully retracted the angiogram showed profuse communication with the biliary tree and contrast within the biliary stents (▶ Fig. 3.150). Superselective embolization of the small lacerated arterial branch of the left hepatic artery and embolization with histoacryl glue (1:4 with Lipiodol) and a 2 × 2 mm detachable microcoil. Postembolization angiogram confirmed lack

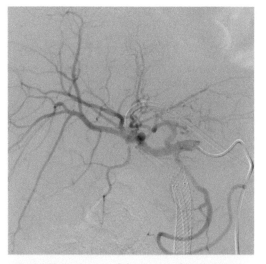

Fig. 3.149 Angiogram of the common hepatic artery with the biliary drain in situ did not show any area of contrast extravasation.

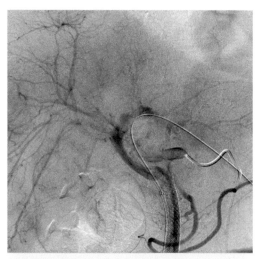

Fig. 3.150 Angiogram of the common hepatic artery when the biliary drain is removed revealed profuse extravasation within the biliary tree with contrast opacification of the biliary stent.

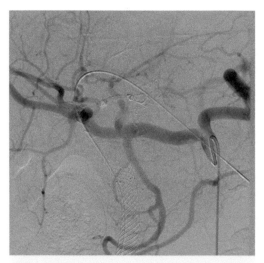

Fig. 3.151 Angiogram of the common hepatic artery after embolization of the small left hepatic artery branch with histoacrylic glue and a coil. No contrast extravasation is detected when the drain is removed.

of opacification of the biliary tree when the drain was removed (▶ Fig. 3.151). The patient remained stable and was discharged 5 days later. He remained free of jaundice in the 2-month follow-up.

Complication Analysis

Laceration of the hepatic artery may occur even when ultrasound guidance for biliary access is used, particularly if a central liver puncture is performed. If the lacerated artery communicates with the biliary tree haemobilia will occur. The laceration needs to be identified early and be managed accordingly. The use of an oversized biliary drain will be effective in sealing bleeding from laceration of a small portal vein branch, but very rarely will resolve an arterial injury that will require embolization. In this particular case the technical difficulty was related to the fact that the extravasation was noted only when the drain was retracted. The drain had to be reinserted immediately in position in order to avoid significant bleeding.

Strategies to Prevent and Take-Home Message

- Use color Doppler ultrasound guidance to avoid the vascular structures of the liver if possible.
- In case of a vessel laceration, try to identify if you are dealing with a low pressure portal vein branch injury of a high flow arterial injury.
- Consider embolization when arterial injury occurs.

Further Reading

Krokidis M, Hatzidakis A. Percutaneous minimally invasive treatment of malignant biliary strictures: current status. Cardiovasc Intervent Radiol. 2014; 37(2):316–323

Choi SH, Gwon DI, Ko GY, et al. Hepatic arterial injuries in 3110 patients following percutaneous transhepatic biliary drainage. Radiology. 2011; 261(3):969–975

Rivera-Sanfeliz GM, Assar OS, LaBerge JM, et al. Incidence of important hemobilia following transhepatic biliary drainage: left-sided versus right-sided approaches. Cardiovasc Intervent Radiol. 2004; 27(2):137–139

Saad WE, Davies MG, Darcy MD. Management of bleeding after percutaneous transhepatic cholangiography or transhepatic biliary drain placement. Tech Vasc Interv Radiol. 2008; 11(1):60–71

3.6.4 Renal Artery Pseudoaneurysm Post Percutaneous Kidney Biopsy

Patient History

A 65-year-old male patient with suspicion of potential interstitial nephritis was referred for percutaneous renal biopsy. No further comorbidities are reported.

Initial Treatment

The patient was scheduled for ultrasound-guided percutaneous renal biopsy (▶ Fig. 3.152) under strict sterility measures; local anesthesia and ultrasound guidance a 16 gauge automatic soft-tissue biopsy needle was inserted and sampling was performed from the lower pole of the left kidney.

Problems Encountered during the Treatment

Unremarkable procedure, no complications reported.

Imaging Plan

One week later patient underwent a chest CT scan (for reasons not related to the biopsy session).

Resulting Complication

A renal pseudoaneurysm is illustrated in the left kidney (▶ Fig. 3.153).

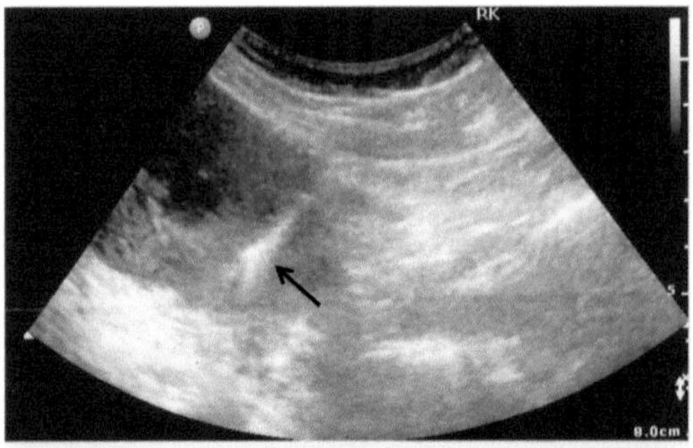

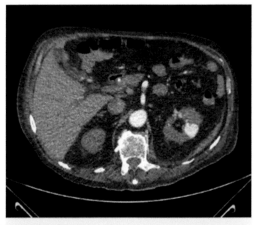

Fig. 3.152 Image taken during the ultrasound guided percutaneous biopsy—needle (*arrow*) is located at left kidney's lower pole.

Fig. 3.153 CT axial scan (postcontrast medium intravenous injection—arterial phase) illustrating the pseudo aneurysm at the lower pole of the left kidney.

What Would You Do?

Notes:

_____

_____

_____

_____

_____

_____

_____

_____

Possible Strategies for Complication Management

- Wait and see approach for spontaneous resolution and closure of the renal pseudoaneurysm.
- Ultrasound-guided percutaneous injection of thrombogenic material.
- Transarterial embolization with thrombogenic agents or occlusive coils.
- Surgery (evacuation and closure of the arterial defect or evacuation and ligation of the offending artery).
- Surgery (nephrectomy).

Final Complication Management

Endovascular treatment via contralateral retrograde access to the common femoral artery (6 French sheath; 5 French angiographic catheter). Catheterization of the feeding vessel by using a microcatheter (2.7 French) followed by selective microcoil embolization (▶ Fig. 3.154).

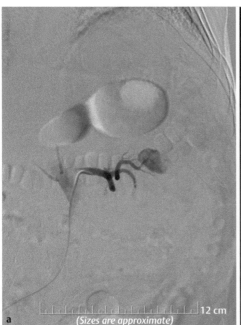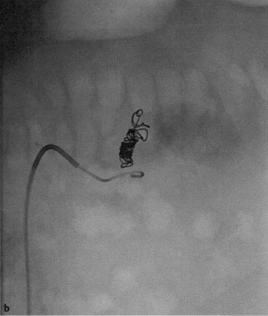

12 cm
(Sizes are approximate)

Fig. 3.154 **(a)** Fluoroscopic view during angiography performed from the 5 French Cobra catheter at the level of the main renal artery—pseudoaneurysm is visible. **(b)** Through the microcatheter (2.7 French) microcoils were already placed.

Complication Analysis

The incidence of renal pseudoaneurysm following percutaneous biopsy is approximately 5%; during the biopsy injury to a branch of the renal artery occurred.

Strategies to Prevent and Take-Home Message

- Whenever patients undergoing renal intervention present with symptoms such as anemia, flank pain and hematuria a high index of suspicion for renal pseudoaneurysm should be prompted.
- Endovascular selective transarterial embolization can be used as first line therapy in cases of renal pseudoaneurysms arising from smaller branches of the renal artery.

- Surgical alternatives can be reserved in cases of renal pseudoaneurysms arising from the main renal artery.
- Decision for management of renal pseudoaneurysms should take account the patient's clinical status along with the therapy's benefits versus the risk of life-threatening hemorrhage.

Further Reading

Guo H, Wang C, Yang M, et al. Management of iatrogenic renal arteriovenous fistula and renal arterial pseudoaneurysm by transarterial embolization: a single center analysis and outcomes. Medicine (Baltimore). 2017; 96(40):e8187

Gonzalez-Aguirre AJ, Durack JC. Managing complications following nephron-sparing procedures for renal masses. Tech Vasc Interv Radiol. 2016; 19(3):194–202

Ngo TC, Lee JJ, Gonzalgo ML. Renal pseudoaneurysm: an overview. Nat Rev Urol. 2010; 7(11):619–625

3.7 Neurologic Event

3.7.1 Complete Motor Deficit of the Lower Limbs during Celiac Plexus Neurolysis

Patient History

A 54-year-old female patient affected by multimetastatic end-stage pancreatic cancer was referred for celiac plexus neurolysis due to persistent upper abdominal pain despite maximal opioid therapy. A pretreatment contrast-enhanced CT scan showed extensive bilateral tumor infiltration of the paravertebral and retrocrural space (▶ Fig. 3.155). A bilateral retrocrural neurolosysis was performed under CT-guidance (▶ Fig. 3.156). The patient was installed in the prone position, following local anesthesia—two 22G spinal needles were bilaterally deployed in the retrocrural space at the level of TH12. Thereafter, 2 mL contrast medium was injected through each needle to check contrast-medium spread in the retrocrural space. Then, 1 mL Xylocaine 1% was injected with each needle, followed by 5 mL of alcohol, 100% on each side. The patient was pain free for the following 10 days, and then she started to experience visceral pain again.

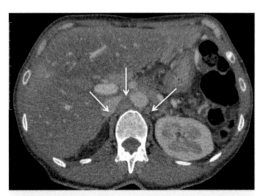

Fig. 3.155 Pretreatment contrast-enhanced CT scan showing extensive bilateral tumor infiltration of the paravertebral and retrocrural space (*arrows*).

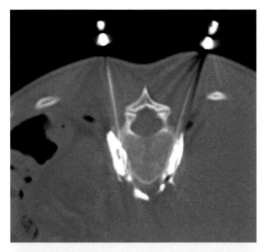

Fig. 3.156 Bilateral retrocrural neurolosysis performed under CT guidance.

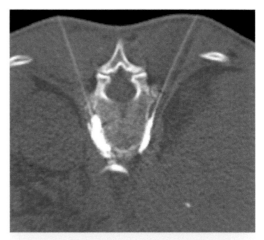

Fig. 3.157 Second bilateral retrocrural neurolosysis performed under CT guidance received by the patient.

Initial Treatment

A new neurolysis was therefore performed with the same aforementioned technique at nearly the same level of TH12 (▶ Fig. 3.157).

Problems Encountered during the Treatment

During injection of contrast medium, the operator felt a slight resistance on the left-sided needle.

Imaging Plan

None.

Resulting Complication

The patient experienced immediate numbness and complete motor deficit of the lower limbs.

What Would You Do?

Notes:

_____

_____

_____

_____

_____

_____

_____

_____

Possible Strategies for Complication Management

- Flushing spinal needles with saline.
- Intravenous fluid replacement and high-dose steroids therapy.
- Conservative management.

Final Complication Management

Both needles were immediately retracted without any further injections and the patient was turned supine and observed until the symptomatology spontaneously resolved within 10 minutes.

Complication Analysis

Celiac plexus neurolysis is a well-established technique for pain management for patients with advanced pancreatic cancer. Major complications have been reported in less than 2% of the cases; in particular, paraplegia has been sporadically reported, and a direct or indirect involvement of the Adamkiewicz artery (i.e., spinal anterior artery) has been advocated as the underlying etiology. Neurologic symptoms may be permanent or more commonly transient; thus, recovering over a variable range of time (minutes–days) either spontaneously, or following adequate intravenous fluid replacement (to maintain adequate blood pressure) and high-dose steroid therapy. The Adamkiewicz artery is the main thoracolumbar artery supplying the anterior two-thirds of the spinal cord. It is always located between TH8 and L3 (50% cases at TH9–TH10 level), and it comes from the left side in 75% of the cases. When blood supply from this artery is compromised, patients rapidly experience complete motor paralysis and loss of pain and temperature sensation at and below the level of injury, autonomic dysfunction (e.g., orthostatic hypotension), and intact proprioception.

The patient presented transitorily reported this symptomatology, thus, configuring a temporary hypoperfusion to the Adamkiewicz artery. The exact etiology of such hypoperfusion is unknown but probably relied on a spasm or a transient compression of the Adamkiewicz artery.

Strategies to Prevent and Take-Home Message

Interestingly, the reported complication occurred just after contrast-medium injection and not following anesthetics or alcohol injection. In fact, in such events, needles should not be removed, and flushing with saline is recommended.

Probably, in the present case, hypoperfusion was provoked by the "high-pressure" injection of contrast medium in a relatively closed and tumor-infiltrated space. Avoidance of such rare complication may be achieved by performing the retrocrural neurolysis at a lower or superior level where tumoral infiltration is less pronounced. Another option may be the anterior approach with neurolytic agents being injected anterolateral to the aorta. Nevertheless, the anterior approach is generally considered less safe since neurolytic agents may spread in the abdominal cavity.

Further Reading

Kambadakone A, Thabet A, Gervais DA, Mueller PR, Arellano RS. CT-guided celiac plexus neurolysis: a review of anatomy, indications, technique, and tips for successful treatment. Radiographics. 2011; 31(6):1599–1621

Arcidiacono PG, Calori G, Carrara S, McNicol ED, Testoni PA. Celiac plexus block for pancreatic cancer pain in adults. Cochrane Database Syst Rev. 2011(3):CD007519

Jabbal SS, Hunton J. Reversible paraplegia following coeliac plexus block. Anaesthesia. 1992; 47(10):857–858

Kumar A, Tripathi SS, Dhar D, Bhattacharya A. A case of reversible paraparesis following celiac plexus block. Reg Anesth Pain Med. 2001; 26(1):75–78

Charles YP, Barbe B, Beaujeux R, Boujan F, Steib JP. Relevance of the anatomical location of the Adamkiewicz artery in spine surgery. Surg Radiol Anat. 2011; 33(1):3–9

Cheshire WP, Santos CC, Massey EW, Howard JF, Jr. Spinal cord infarction: etiology and outcome. Neurology. 1996; 47(2):321–330

3.7.2 Nontarget Embolization during Transarterial Chemoembolization for Hepatocellular Carcinoma Treatment: Be Aware of the Arteria Radicularis Magna

Patient History

A 52-year-old affected from cirrhosis was presented with a 17.5 × 12.3 cm hepatocellular carcinoma occupying nearly the whole of the right liver lobe with portal vein invasion and presence of arterioportal shunts and extrahepatic arterial supply (▶ Fig. 3.158). The lesion was considered as inoperable and treatment with transarterial chemoembolization was decided by the multidisciplinary team meeting.

Initial Treatment

The patient received multiple sessions of superselective transarterial chemoembolization with the use of lipiodol, in a 3-year period. During the first chemoembolization sessions the presence of arterioportal shunts was confirmed (▶ Fig. 3.159) that was slightly reduced after the sixth treatment session (▶ Fig. 3.160). The patient's clinical condition has significantly improved during this course of treatment.

Problems Encountered during Treatment

Due to the large size of the lesion extra hepatic feeders via the intercostal arteries had to be

identified in the next superselective transarterial chemoembolization sessions (▶ Fig. 3.161). For the 10th embolization session another intercostal feeder was catheterized. However, the intercostal feeder communicated with the anterior spinal artery (or arteria radicularis magna or artery of

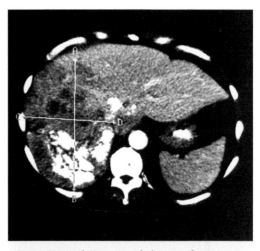

Fig. 3.158 Initial CT in arterial phase, confirming a 17.5 × 12.3 cm hepatocellular carcinoma occupying the whole right liver lobe.

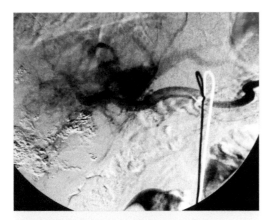

Fig. 3.159 Coeliac axis arteriogram reveals the presence of extensive arterioportal shunts during the initial conventional transarterial chemoembolization.

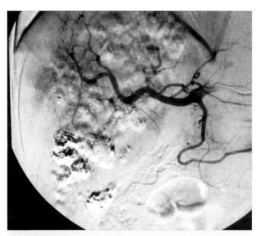

Fig. 3.160 Hepatic angiogram after six conventional transarterial chemoembolization sessions, confirming reduction of the arterioportal shunt.

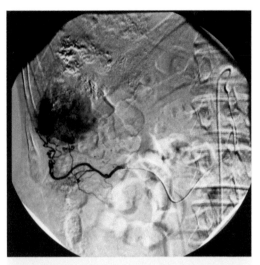

Fig. 3.161 Superselective catheterization of an intercostal artery revealed the arterial supply to the lesion. Conventional transarterial chemoembolization from that position followed.

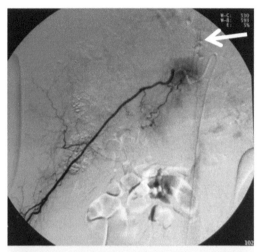

Fig. 3.162 Superselective catheterization of an intercostal artery of a different level. The arteria a radicularis magna (*arrow*) was detected at the final angiograms due to the decrease of flow velocity. Reflux of the embolization material in the artery accidentally occurred.

Ademkiewicz). The artery was not identified at the first angiogram due to the predilection of the flow toward the lesion. When the embolization reduced the flow in the lesion and the flow was slower, the artery became visible angiographically (▶ Fig. 3.162). Nontarget embolization in the artery at that stage was inevitable due to reflux of the embolic material. The patient developed immediate paraplegia and urine incontinence. He passed away 1.5 years later due to advanced disease. His total survival after diagnosis was 50 months.

Imaging Plan

A spinal MRI may be performed to assess the extension of the ischemic damage.

Resulting Complication

Paraplegia due to nontarget embolization in the arteria radicularis magna.

Complication Analysis

The prevalence of right lumbar artery supply to the hepatocellular carcinoma (HCC) has been reported around 2%. Usually, patients undergo a number of chemoembolization sessions before the blood supply from the intercostal arteries is discovered. The intercostal supply may be related to a damage of the main hepatic supply; however, this is not a necessary condition. In such cases arteriograms of the right lower intercostal arteries (TH10 and TH11), the subcostal artery, and the right upper lumbar arteries (L1 and L2) need to be performed to determine where the origin of the anterior spinal artery is. Nontarget embolization of the anterior spinal artery is a dramatic complication because has an immediate and irreversible effect.

From what is reported in the literature when the anterior spinal artery is not taking origin from the catheterized lumbar artery or adjacent arteries, chemoembolization followed by gelatin sponge particles is performed. When the anterior spinal artery takes origin from the tumor-feeding branch or any of the adjacent arteries, then embolization with gelatin sponge particles alone is suggested.

In this case the large size of the lesion implemented embolization via the small intercostal feeders, which is usually rare for medium size HCCs. The artery could not be identified at the initial stage of the procedure because of the forward flow toward the lesion. However, it needs to be taken into account that the origin of the artery is usually in the proximal third of the intercostal and super selective catheterization in a more distal position needs is a more secure approach. Furthermore, given that reflux may occur even from a more distal position, the use of larger size particles (>300 µm) may reduce the risk of nontarget embolization.

Strategies to Prevent and Take-Home Message

- Keep in mind that there is communication of the anterior spinal artery with intercostal arteries.
- The artery can only be identified when the flow is slow at the end of the embolization session.

- Aim to be more selective in such cases.
- Use microparticles of large size (>300 µm) and there will be small chances of reflux.

Further Reading

Kim HC, Chung JW, Lee W, Jae HJ, Park JH. Recognizing extrahepatic collateral vessels that supply hepatocellular carcinoma to avoid complications of transcatheter arterial chemoembolization. Radiographics. 2005; 25 Suppl 1:S25–S39

Miyayama S, Yamashiro M, Okuda M, et al. Hepatocellular carcinoma supplied by the right lumbar artery. Cardiovasc Intervent Radiol. 2010; 33(1):53–60

Miyayama S, Matsui O, Taki K, et al. Transcatheter arterial chemoembolization for hepatocellular carcinoma fed by the reconstructed inferior phrenic artery: anatomical and technical analysis. J Vasc Interv Radiol. 2004; 15(8):815–823

3.8 Pneumothorax

3.8.1 Delayed Pneumothorax after Lung Biopsy

Patient History

A 61-year-old female, with history of asthma and chronic obstructive pulmonary disease (COPD), was scheduled for CT-guided right lung biopsy.

Initial Treatment

CT-guided biopsy of the right lung lesion was performed using an 18 gauge coaxial biopsy system (▶ Fig. 3.163, ▶ Fig. 3.164). Four core needle samples of the right upper lobe nodule were obtained. Post-procedure images were acquired, without any evidence of pneumothorax.

Problems Encountered during the Treatment

The patient tolerated the procedure without any complication and was subsequently transferred to the recovery unit in stable condition.

Imaging Plan

A follow-up chest radiograph was scheduled for 2 hours later.

Resulting Complication

The patient developed chest pain approximately 1 hour after the procedure. Decreased breathing sounds were noted in the right hemithorax on physical examination. The follow-up chest radiograph revealed a large right pneumothorax (▶ Fig. 3.165).

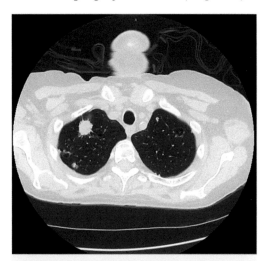

Fig. 3.163 Contrast-enhanced CT scan of chest demonstrates a speculated pulmonary nodule in the right upper lobe before biopsy.

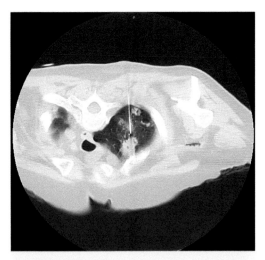

Fig. 3.164 CT-guided percutaneous biopsy of the right upper lobe nodule is performed through right paravertebral approach, while the patient is placed in prone position.

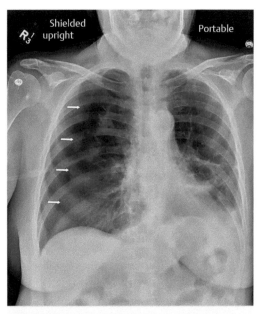

Fig. 3.165 The post-procedural chest radiography reveals a large right pneumothorax.

What Would You Do?

Notes:

_____

_____

_____

_____

_____

_____

_____

_____

Possible Strategies for Complication Management

- Conservative treatment.
- CT versus fluoroscopic-guided chest tube placement.

Final Complication Management

Under fluoroscopic guidance, a small caliber needle was advanced into the pleural space and aspirated. Then, a 10 French chest tube was placed into the right pleural space, connected to a Pneumovac.

Complication Analysis

A small pneumothorax developed during the procedure. However, the pneumothorax expanded post-procedure in the observation unit, causing chest pain.

Strategies to Prevent and Take-Home Message

- Respiration instruction and advancing the needle after exhalation could reduce the risk of pneumothorax.
- Minimizing number of pleural puncture.
- Patients with COPD and emphysema have increased risk of developing a post-procedural pneumothorax.
- Avoid using needles larger than 20 gauge, as they put the patient at increased risk of pneumothorax and hemothorax.
- Obtain final images immediately after removal of the needle. Observe patient's vital sign for 2 to 4 hours following the procedure (▶ Fig. 3.166).

Further Reading

Boskovic T, Stanic J, Pena-Karan S, et al. Pneumothorax after transthoracic needle biopsy of lung lesions under CT guidance. J Thorac Dis. 2014; 6 Suppl 1:S99–S107

Choi CM, Um SW, Yoo CG, et al. Incidence and risk factors of delayed pneumothorax after transthoracic needle biopsy of the lung. Chest. 2004; 126(5):1516–1521

Topal U, Ediz B. Transthoracic needle biopsy: factors effecting risk of pneumothorax. Eur J Radiol. 2003; 48(3):263–267

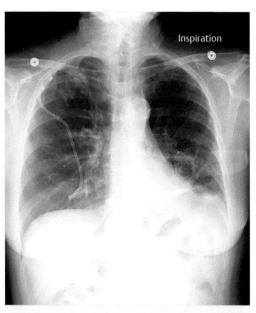

Inspiration

Fig. 3.166 The chest radiography demonstrates the chest tube terminating in the right upper hemithorax with complete resolution of pneumothorax.

3.8.2 Pneumothorax during Microwave Ablation for Treatment of a Single Pulmonary Metastasis

Patient History

A 68-year-old male patient underwent microwave ablation (MWA) for the treatment of a single pulmonary metastasis located in the lower lobe of the left lung (▶ Fig. 3.167). The underlying tumor was a colorectal adenocarcinoma. He had previous coronary stenting procedure for myocardial infarction treatment without any other comorbidity. He underwent four cycles of chemotherapy, resulting only in small reduction of the pulmonary lesion size.

Initial Treatment

Percutaneous MWA was performed under real-time CT guidance and under conscious sedation with the patient in lateral position on the right side. The access route was 10 French.

Problems Encountered during the Treatment and Imaging Plan

During the treatment a pneumothorax occurred, displacing the lesion very closely to the aorta (▶ Fig. 3.168, ▶ Fig. 3.169).

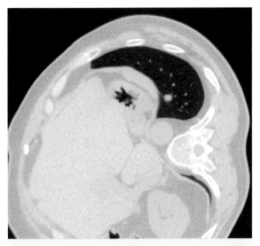

Fig. 3.167 CT scan in lung window shows a 7 mm round nodule in the medial segment of the left lower lobe already diagnosed as metastasis. Note that the lesion is close to the diaphragm but far about 3 cm from the descending aorta.

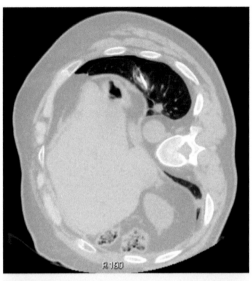

Fig. 3.168 CT scan demonstrates a pneuomothorax following placement of the microwave antenna. Note that pneumothorax caused resulted to a partial collapse of the lung and displaced the lesion close to the aorta.

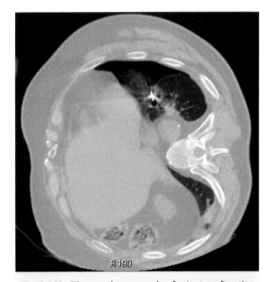

Fig. 3.169 CT scan taken a couple of minutes after the previous image shows either the worsening pneumothorax or an even more important collapse of the lung attaching the nodule to the paramediastinal pleura and making the attempts of lesion targeting difficult and risky.

What Would You Do?

Notes:

_____

_____

_____

_____

_____

_____

_____

_____

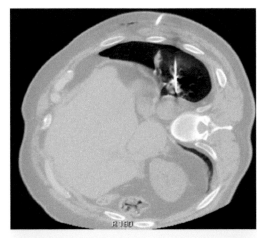

Fig. 3.170 CT scan showing the microwave antenna's tip inside the lesion, after lung re-expansion. Note the subcutaneous tract of pigtail catheter used for pleural drainage.

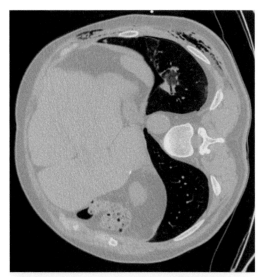

Fig. 3.171 Post-procedural CT scan demonstrates the results of microwave ablation with findings of subcutaneous emphysema.

Possible Strategies for Complication Management

- Procedure suspension and thoracic drainage.
- Percutaneous drainage.

Final Complication Management

The pneumothorax was treated with a percutaneous thoracic drainage (10 French pig-tail catheter); it ensured a lung expansion and allowed to follow with the MWA (► Fig. 3.170). The chest tube remained in place for 48 hours, and then it was removed (► Fig. 3.171); the patient was discharged home doing well at day 3 after the procedure.

Complication Analysis

Even if the patient had no risk factors for pneumothorax like emphysema, the pulmonary lesion was small, deep, and very close to the diaphragm. The increased distance traversed is an important risk factor for major complications like pneumothorax; however, we preferred a lateral approach with the patient in lateral position to allow a more comfortable anesthesiologist approach and to avoid risky puncture of diaphragm with the tip of the microwave antenna.

Strategies to Prevent and Take-Home Message

Although MWA for lung cancer is a safe procedure, it may cause significant complications like pneumothorax. Precautions to minimize risk factors should be taken, if possible, and of course the team must be experienced in immediate drainage placement. As a general rule, in particular in males and advanced age patients it is very important to reduce the length of the treated lung traversed by the antenna.

Further Reading

Splatt AM, Steinke K. Major complications of high-energy microwave ablation for percutaneous CT-guided treatment of lung malignancies: single-centre experience after 4 years. J Med Imaging Radiat Oncol. 2015; 59(5):609–616

Carrafiello G, Mangini M, Fontana F, et al. Complications of microwave and radiofrequency lung ablation: personal experience and review of the literature. Radiol Med (Torino). 2012; 117(2): 201–213

Zheng A, Wang X, Yang X, et al. Major complications after lung microwave ablation: a single-center experience on 204 sessions. Ann Thorac Surg. 2014; 98(1):243–248

3.8.3 Pneumothorax during Diagnostic CT-Guided Lung Puncture

Patient History

An 82-year-old male patient with 25 mm lesion of the right lung, peripheral located (segment 4), was scheduled for CT-guided diagnostic puncture in order to obtain the exact diagnosis; bronchial carcinoma was suspected. Laboratory blood tests indicated neither compromised coagulation parameters, nor any pathologic blood count.

Initial Treatment

So far no treatment was done. The diagnostic procedure was planned for further diagnostic reasons in order to offer the patient an individualized treatment concept.

Diagnostic puncture was done under local anesthesia with 10 mL Prilocaine hydrochloride 1%. The body was elevated for 80 degrees to the left side in order to start percutaneous access in the posterior axillary line. After the skin incision, 16G 6 cm

Trokar (Quick-Core Biopsy Needle Set, Cook, Bloomington, IN, USA) was inserted and after checking the adequate position, an 18G 9 cm biopsy needle was inserted, and 5 probes were successfully taken (▶ Fig. 3.172).

Problems Encountered during the Treatment

After the last probe, the control scan before removing the trocar showed pneumothorax (▶ Fig. 3.173). The patient was fully compensated.

Imaging Plan

Completing thorax CT scan to determine the exact size of pneumothorax.

Resulting Complication

Pneumothorax appearance during diagnostic peripheral lung puncture.

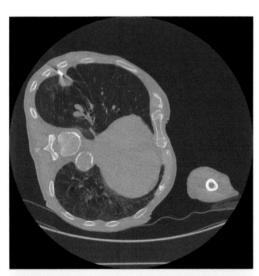

Fig. 3.172 Native axial CT scan of the right lung showing a 25 mm tumor-like subpleural lesion located in segment 4 with corresponding pleural thickening. The trocar is already in place ready for inserting the biopsy needle.

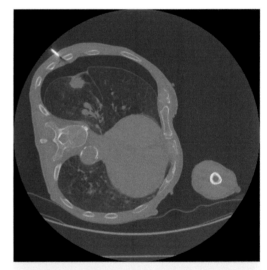

Fig. 3.173 CT after five biopsies and partially retracted trocar. A significant pneumothorax is visible.

What Would You Do?

Notes:

_____

_____

_____

_____

_____

_____

_____

_____

Possible Strategies for Complication Management

- Suction via trocar with a 50 cc syringe.
- Placement of an intermediate drainage (Bülau, Moldini).
- Leave it as it is (if the patient is fully compensated).

Final Complication Management

Drainage insertion done by the thoracic surgeons.

Complication Analysis

During puncture and biopsy, pneumothorax occurred. Reasons for that may be due to trocar dislocation during movement/forced in and expiration. Repeated manipulation such as removing and advancing a biopsy needle through the trocar might be responsible for pleural injury resulting in pneumothorax.

Strategies to Prevent and Take-Home Message

- Handle instruments with care. Try to focus on peripheral located lesions. More central lesions are prone for complications like pneumothorax and haemoptoe.
- Chronic obstructive pulmonary disease patients are prone for complications as described, avoid the biopsy them percutaneously.
- Try to limit the size of your trocar to 16G (as done in the introductory case).

Further Reading

Heerink WJ, de Bock GH, de Jonge GJ, Groen HJM, Vliegenthart R, Oudkerk M. Complication rates of CT-guided transthoracic lung biopsy: meta-analysis. Eur Radiol. 2017; 27(1):138–148

Digumarthy SR, Kovacina B, Otrakji A, Lanuti M, Shepard JA, Sharma A. Percutaneous CT guided lung biopsy in patients with pulmonary hypertension: assessment of complications. Eur J Radiol. 2016; 85(2):466–471

Galluzzo A, Genova C, Dioguardi S, Midiri M, Cajozzo M. Current role of computed tomography-guided transthoracic needle biopsy of metastatic lung lesions. Future Oncol. 2015; 11(2) Suppl:43–46

3.8.4 Intraprocedural Pneumothorax after Biopsy before Microwave Ablation

Patient History

A 68-year-old female current smoker with history of right upper lobe squamous cell cancer (SCC) 6 years prior and SCC of the cervix 14 years prior, both treated with chemoradiotherapy, presented with a growing speculated FDG-PET avid middle lobe nodule infiltrating the oblique fissure (▶ Fig. 3.174) for consideration of treatment options.

Initial Treatment and Imaging Plan

Thermal ablation was thought to be the appropriate treatment. Tissue diagnosis was sought; a CT-guided core biopsy was planned to be performed immediately prior to microwave ablation. Using a coaxial approach, two passes with a Bard Mission 20G core biopsy needle 20 mm (Tempe, Arizona, USA) were performed.

Resulting Complication

A pneumothorax occurred during biopsy, which enlarged upon withdrawal of the biopsy needle (▶ Fig. 3.175).

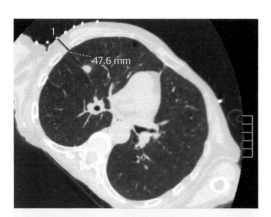

Fig. 3.174 Axial CT lung window shows the spiculated middle lobe nodule infiltrating the oblique fissure. Skin marker and planned biopsy/ablation trajectory drawn.

What Would You Do?
Notes:

Possible Strategies for Complication Management

- Abort and reschedule for thermal ablation.
- Abort and reschedule for thermal ablation, insert a pigtail catheter/chest tube.
- Abort and reschedule for thermal ablation after aspirating air from the pleural space through the coaxial needle or any other small bore catheter (e.g., venous cannula).
- Attempt aspiration of the air and continue with ablation if successful.

Final Complication Management

An extension tube with a 3-way tap was connected to the hub of the coaxial needle and the free air was aspirated. The microwave antenna (standard

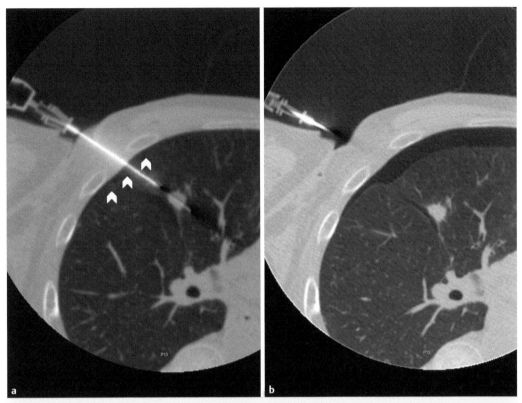

Fig. 3.175 **(a)** Coaxial needle (19 gauge) and matching core biopsy needle (20 gauge) in situ; small pneumothorax at the needle entry site (*arrowheads*). **(b)** Pneumothorax has enlarged upon withdrawal of the biopsy needle, air also in the interlobar fissure. Note that biopsy revealed metachronous SCC.

1.8 mm Accu2i pMTA applicator, AngioDynamics, Queensbury, NY, USA) was inserted parallel to the coaxial needle (▶ Fig. 3.176) and the ablation was performed as planned, intermittently aspirating air to keep the lung inflated and prevent unintended thermal damage of adjacent pulmonary parenchyma.

The immediate postablation CT scan after removal of the ablation device and the coaxial needle showed only a tiny residual pneumothorax in the interlobar fissure the target nodule was abutting (▶ Fig. 3.177). The 24-hour CT scan showed the intended circumferential thermal damage (▶ Fig. 3.177, inset) along with an anterior atelectatic component and slightly enlarged pneumothorax, which remained asymptomatic, did not require aspiration, and resolved spontaneously.

Complication Analysis, Strategies to Prevent, and Take-Home Message

- Pneumothorax is a frequent complication with lung interventions and often unpreventable, even when following recommendation for safe access.
- Pneumothorax seldom precludes successful lung biopsy or ablation.
- Pneumothorax happens in more than 95% of cases while patient still on CT table with interventionalist able to take immediate measures—(repeat) aspiration or insertion of catheter or thoracic vent if lung keeps collapsing.
- With the mismatch of coaxial needle size for biopsy (19G) and microwave applicator size (1.8 mm, approximately 14G), a 13G coaxial

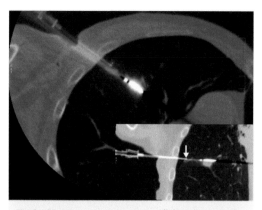

Fig. 3.176 Microwave antenna parallel to the coaxial needle; antenna within the target lesion through the superior third of the nodule, tip of coaxial needle in the pleural space (*white arrow* inset, paracoronal reformat).

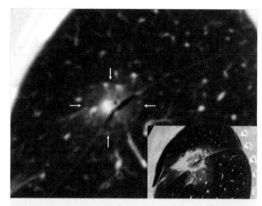

Fig. 3.177 Sagittal reformat lung window immediately post ablation shows the small residual pneumothorax in the interlobar fissure and a rim of faint circumferential surrounding ground-glass opacity around the ablated nodule. The 24-hour image (inset) depicts the surrounding thermal damage and an enlarged pneumothorax.

needle would be necessary to accommodate both the biopsy needle and the ablation device, which is not ideal for the biopsy setting and bears the risk of causing air embolism, hence the biopsy equipment should be removed before the ablation device is inserted.

- It is worth attempting to aspirate the pneumothorax and aim for continuing with the planned intervention; at times a small pneumothorax is a welcome complication with peripherally located lesions, preventing thermal damage to the visceral pleura or chest wall.
- Unresolved pneumothorax is often a sign of bronchopleural fistula.

Further Reading

Lee EW, Suh RD, Zeidler MR, et al. Radiofrequency ablation of subpleural lung malignancy: reduced pain using an artificially created pneumothorax. Cardiovasc Intervent Radiol. 2009; 32 (4):833–836

Nour-Eldin NE, Naguib NN, Tawfik AM, Koitka K, Saeed AS, Vogl TJ. Outcomes of an algorithmic approach to management of pneumothorax complicating thermal ablation of pulmonary neoplasms. J Vasc Interv Radiol. 2011; 22(9):1279–1286

Yamagami T, Kato T, Hirota T, Yoshimatsu R, Matsumoto T, Nishimura T. Usefulness and limitation of manual aspiration immediately after pneumothorax complicating interventional radiological procedures with the transthoracic approach. Cardiovasc Intervent Radiol. 2006; 29(6):1027–1033

3.8.5 Pneumothorax after Percutaneous Lung Interstitial Brachytherapy in Solitary Colorectal Adenocarcinoma Metastasis

Patient History

An 85-year-old male patient presented with a solitary lung metastasis of the underlying rectal cancer in the left lower lobe. Primary origin was confirmed by biopsy. After rectal surgery, and chemoradiation the only site of persistent and progressive malignancy was the target lesion in the lung (▶ Fig. 3.178). Because the first operation

compromised the patient, he refused further surgery. To achieve save margins in this borderline sized lesion we decided to perform an interstitial high-dose-rate brachytherapy (iHDR BT) instead of thermal ablation. Because the aim of iHDR BT is not to destroy the target tissue during the intervention, rather it is turned into necrosis approximately in the following 6 weeks, the risk potential of the

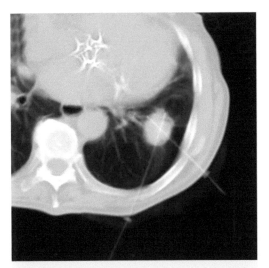

Fig. 3.178 Axial CT scan showing target lesion pierced by percutaneous applicators carrying Iridium (Ir 192).

intervention is comparable to a biopsy. However, every percutaneous manipulation of the lung carries the risk of pneumothorax (3.1% in biopsy).

Initial Treatment

CT-guided interstitial high-dose rate brachytherapy of the lung (▶ Fig. 3.179).

Problems Encountered during the Treatment

Significant pneumothorax was noticed during a control scan after removal of the applicators (▶ Fig. 3.180). Otherwise the procedure was unremarkable, no complications were apparent.

Imaging Plan

Nonenhanced computed tomography of the chest was done on a regular base.

Resulting Complication

Pneumothorax at the site of puncture.

Possible Strategies for Complication Management

- Wait and see in case of limited pneumothorax.
- Chest tube insertion.
- Surgery (if chest tube fails).

Final Complication Management

Chest tube insertion, resulting in complete expansion of the lung (▶ Fig. 3.181).

Complication Analysis

iHDR BT of a lung malignancy resulted in a pneumothorax.

Strategies to Prevent and Take-Home Message

- Lung interventions basically carry the risk of a pneumothorax.
- Radiologists should always follow-up with patients after pulmonary interventions to be able to provide required acute care (▶ Fig. 3.182).

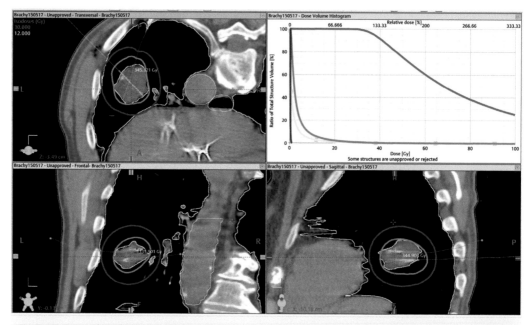

Fig. 3.179 Dose volume histogram: the target lesion had a volume of 14.84 cm³, thus 0.36% of the volume of the entire lung (4,080; 48 cm³). The therapeutic 30 Gy (*red border strip*) were applied in a volume of 24.33 cm³ (0.84% of the lung volume) encircling the target lesion. The blue border strip marks the 12 Gy-isodose (126.77 cm³; 3.1% of the lung volume).

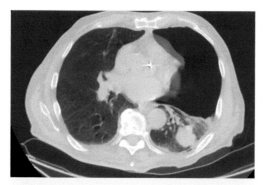

Fig. 3.180 Axial CT scan after removal of the two applicators a significant, ipsilateral pneumothorax occurred.

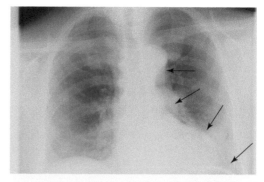

Fig. 3.181 X-ray after introduction of a chest tube a rapid expansion of the collapsed lung could be achieved.

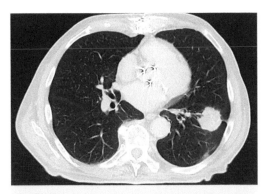

Fig. 3.182 Complete expansion of the lung after removal of the chest drain confirmed by CT. Only local parenchymal hematoma on the sites of the applicators is visible.

Further Reading

Lorenz J, Blum M. Complications of percutaneous chest biopsy. Semin Intervent Radiol. 2006; 23(2):188–193

Sharma DN, Rath GK, Thulkar S, Bahl A, Pandit S, Julka PK. Computerized tomography-guided percutaneous high-dose-rate interstitial brachytherapy for malignant lung lesions. J Cancer Res Ther. 2011; 7(2):174–179

Tselis N, Ferentinos K, Kolotas C, et al. Computed tomography-guided interstitial high-dose-rate brachytherapy in the local treatment of primary and secondary intrathoracic malignancies. J Thorac Oncol. 2011; 6(3):545–552

de Baère T, Aupérin A, Deschamps F, et al. Radiofrequency ablation is a valid treatment option for lung metastases: experience in 566 patients with 1037 metastases. Ann Oncol. 2015; 26(5): 987–991

Ridge CA, Solomon SB. Percutaneous ablation of colorectal lung metastases. J Gastrointest Oncol. 2015; 6(6):685–692

3.9 Skin Burn

3.9.1 Skin Burn after Radiofrequency Ablation of Lung Nodule

Patient History

A 57-year-old female patient with history of advanced non-small cell lung cancer post-chemoradiotherapy of recurrent left lower lobe lung primary and metastasectomy of right lung was discussed interdisciplinary for further treatment. New right lower lobe lung nodule (▶ Fig. 3.183) was scheduled for thermal ablation.

Initial Treatment and Imaging Plan

The patient was scheduled for CT-guided radiofrequency ablation (RFA). Prone position was chosen.

Analgesia and sedation was taken care of by the anesthetic team. A Cool-tip RFA single electrode (Metronic; Minneapolis, MN, USA; with a 2 cm active tip was inserted via a paraspinal access (▶ Fig. 3.184a).

Problems Encountered during the Treatment

A small intra-procedural pneumothorax occurred, moving the target lesion with the electrode in situ slightly inward. The tip of the electrode was very close to an adjacent vessel with the risk of probe migration and vessel injury causing hemorrhage. The electrode was pulled back by 2 to 3 mm and a straight metal forceps was positioned across the electrode shaft at the skin level to prevent the electrode from inadvertent displacement (▶ Fig. 3.184b).

Resulting Complication

Burning smell prompted checking of the electrode entry site; the skin showed focal redness and blistering. The clamp was removed and the ablation cycle continued.

By the end of the ablation a third degree skin burn had occurred (▶ Fig. 3.185a). CT scan postablation (▶ Fig. 3.185b) shows skin thickening and linear burn site through chest wall. The insulation of the electrode has been breached by the sharp serrated metal clamp, leading to propagation of the electric current along the electrode shaft and subsequently into and along the forceps.

Final Complication Management

The patient was referred to the burns team; debridement was necessary.

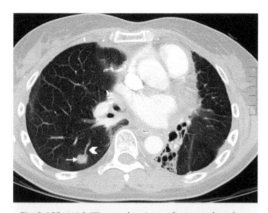

Fig. 3.183 Axial CT scan showing radiation induced traction bronchiectasis medially in the left lower lobe, surgical clips at the right hilum and suture material from linear mechanical stapler anteriorly in right paracardial location from metastasectomy. New right lower lobe of 12 mm solid nodule (*arrow*) with anteriorly abutting vessel is visible (*arrowhead*).

Strategies to Prevent and Take-Home Message

- Use plastic clamps or wrap gauze or other fabric around the electrode shaft if using metal forceps. Be aware that patients under deep analog sedation will not react appropriately to pain stimuli.
- Check electrode/antenna position occasionally during ablation cycle (e.g., with fluoroscopy–CT) to ensure stable intra-procedural findings.
- The use of metal coaxial needles should also be done with caution and the introductory needle withdrawn after positioning of the active electrode to avoid contact with or proximity to the active tip.
- Skin burns related to percutaneous thermal ablations have mainly been reported at the site of indifferent electrode/grounding pad in lengthy and complex RFA cases.
- Case reports of skin burns at the interstitial electrode entry sites have been described with superficial ablations (e.g., bone and thyroid).

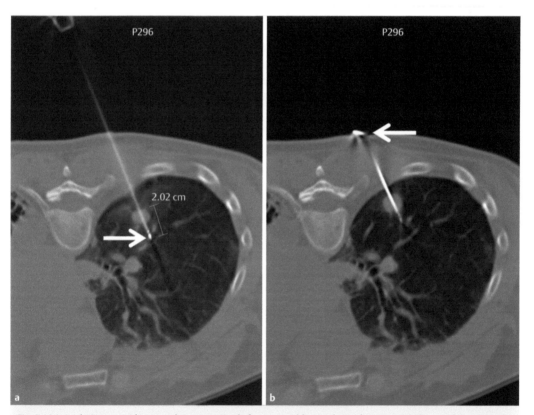

Fig. 3.184 Axial CT scans with patient lying prone, radiofrequency ablation electrode in situ. **(a)** The tip of the electrode running centrally through the target lesion is abutting the medium sized anterior vessel (*arrow*). **(b)** The electrode has been retracted by a few millimeters and a straight metal forceps placed across the electrode shaft (*arrow*).

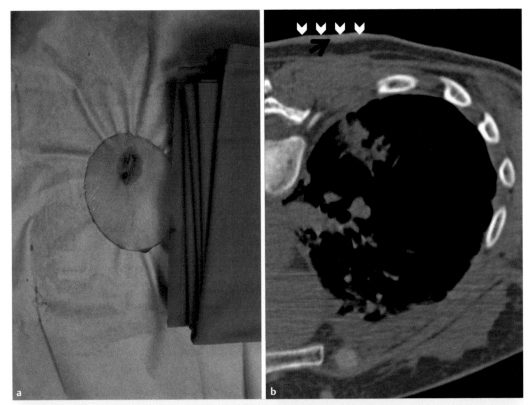

Fig. 3.185 (a) The image showing third-degree skin burn at the site where the metal forceps was in contact with the skin. **(b)** Axial CT scan intermediate window with *white arrowheads* delineating the area of skin thickening; faint dark line (*black arrow*) through the thickened skin denoting the track of the electrode along which the burn has occurred.

Further Reading

Steinke K, Gananadha S, King J, Zhao J, Morris DL. Dispersive pad site burns with modern radiofrequency ablation equipment. Surg Laparosc Endosc Percutan Tech. 2003; 13(6):366–371

Liang P, Wang Y, Yu X, Dong B. Malignant liver tumors: treatment with percutaneous microwave ablation—complications among cohort of 1136 patients. Radiology. 2009; 251(3):933–940

Bernardi S, Lanzilotti V, Papa G, et al. Full-thickness skin burn caused by radiofrequency ablation of a benign thyroid nodule. Thyroid. 2016; 26(1):183–184

Widmann G, Jaschke W, Bale R. Case report: third-degree skin and soft tissue burn after radiofrequency ablation of an osteoid osteoma guided through a triple-crown biopsy cannula. Skeletal Radiol. 2012; 41(12):1627–1630

3.9.2 Burned Skin after Radiofrequency Ablation for Osteoid Osteoma Treatment

Patient History

A 27-year-old female patient with 9 mm cortical lesion of the anterior tibia diaphysis and the typical clinical history of pain was scheduled for thermal ablation. Diagnostic X-ray (▶ Fig. 3.186) showed a cortical thickening and axial CT as well as the sagittal reconstruction presented an oval lesion with a hypodense nidus located in the anterior tibia (▶ Fig. 3.187, ▶ Fig. 3.188).

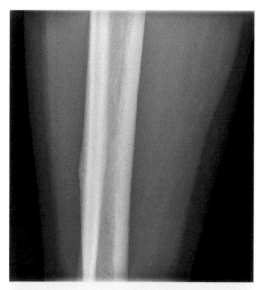

Fig. 3.186 X-ray of the tibial bone showing an ellipsoid thickening of the corticalis indicating the underlying lesion.

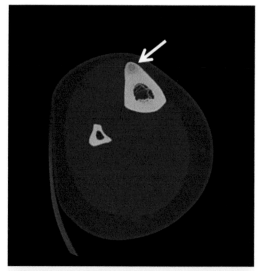

Fig. 3.187 Axial CT presenting the lesion with a central, more hypodense area representing the nidus (*arrow*). Note the thin subcutaneous covering of the bone resulting in a rather short distance to the skin.

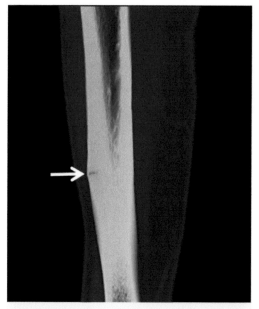

Fig. 3.188 Sagittal reconstruction of the tibia diaphysis indicting the lesion with the nidus (*arrow*).

Initial Treatment

The ablation procedure was planned under general anesthesia and after ski disinfection and incision; a 1.8 mm K-wire drill was used to get access to the lesion. The radiofrequency electrode was inserted through the drill track into the osteoid osteoma and confirmed with CT. For radiofrequency ablation (RFA) a 16.5G, 18 cm Soloist-single needle electrode (active electrode 0.9 mm; Boston Scientific Corporation, Natick, MA, USA) was placed in the lesion. A radiofrequency of 3,000 Generator corresponding to the needle, with impedance-based feedback system and 200 W capacity was activated after placement of a proper grounding pads were placed on both upper legs to reduce risk of complications. RFA was started according the instruction or use.

Problems Encountered during the Treatment

No problems during the procedure were noted.

Imaging Plan

Routine MRI was scheduled for day one after the procedure showing typical post-procedure findings with some moderate contrast enhancement of the subcutaneous tissue, the epifascial tissue and the channel towards the lesion and at the lesion itself (▶ Fig. 3.189).

Resulting Complication

Skin was noted erythematous with second degree thermal burn followed by development of skin necrosis within the next days.

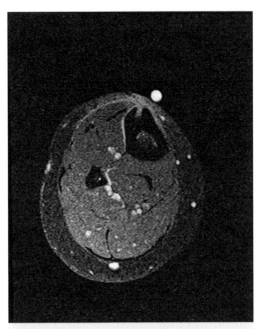

Fig. 3.189 Contrast-enhanced MRI (T1, fat suppressed) showing the burr channel, the lesion and the subcutaneous tissue with intense signal representing contrast enhancing. A signal intense outer capsule indicates the former skin entrance level.

What Would You Do?

Notes:

_____

_____

_____

_____

_____

_____

_____

Possible Strategies for Complication Management

- Skin cooling during initial treatment.

Final Complication Management

Surgical skin revision and wound closure.

Complication Analysis

During RFA of a bone lesion, skin injury/burn occurred. A thin subcutaneous tissue a lesion site was burned due to the nonisolated electrode and short access channel. Areas at greatest risk are those without much subcutaneous fat or muscle, such as the anterior tibia.

Strategies to Prevent and Take-Home Message

- Choose a different access route with a thicker tissue covering.
- Guarantee adequate cooling of the superficial tissue at needle entrance site.

Further Reading

Huffman SD, Huffman NP, Lewandowski RJ, Brown DB. Radiofrequency ablation complicated by skin burn. Semin Intervent Radiol. 2011; 28(2):179–182

Lyon C, Buckwalter J. Case report: full-thickness skin necrosis after percutaneous radio-frequency ablation of a tibial osteoid osteoma. Iowa Orthop J. 2008; 28:85–87

Finstein JL, Hosalkar HS, Ogilvie CM, Lackman RD. Case reports: an unusual complication of radiofrequency ablation treatment of osteoid osteoma. Clin Orthop Relat Res. 2006; 448 (448):248–251

3.9.3 Skin Burn after Dislocation of a Microwave Ablation Electrode during Ablation of Liver Metastases in Coaxial Technique

Patient History

A 70-year-old male patient in good general clinical condition was diagnosed with CCC of the liver involving segments 2/3 of the left lobe. A 3 cm intrahepatic metastasis was located in segment 5. Otherwise the patient was tumor free.

Initial Treatment

Tumor board consensus recommended the following treatment strategy: (1) operative resection of the main tumor followed by (2) locoregional therapy of the remaining metastasis in segment 5 (▶ Fig. 3.190).

For ablation, four true-guide 14 French coaxial needles (Bard, Murray Hill, NJ, USA) were placed in the periphery of the tumor to facilitate A0 ablation with sufficient margins. Needle tips had a distance of 1.5 cm from each other. In coaxial technique 2 14 French Syncrowave antenna (Medtronic; Minneapolis, MN, USA) were inserted in two of the coaxial needles for a run of ablation for the anterior aspect of the tumor. Before ablation the coaxial needles were retracted as far back to the skin entry point as possible to avoid thermal damage (▶ Fig. 3.191). The two unused coaxial

metal needles, which were planned to host the antennas for a second ablation run remained in the dorsal aspect of the tumor neighboring the active antennas.

Problems Encountered during the Treatment

During ablation with 90 W for 12 minutes, tissue swelling around the needle entry points occurred. Contrast-enhanced CT control following the first microwave ablation (MWA) run showed hypoattenuation of the liver reaching the capsule in combination with thickening, fluid and air accumulation in the abdominal wall, consistent with thermal damage. The procedure was not continued.

Resulting Complication

Peripheral liver necrosis and thermal damage to the abdominal wall (▶ Fig. 3.192). Incomplete ablation of the metastasis.

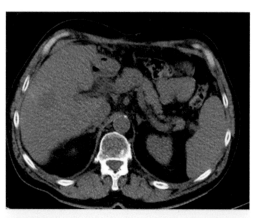

Fig. 3.190 Native CT showing a 3 cm hypodense mass in the right lobe.

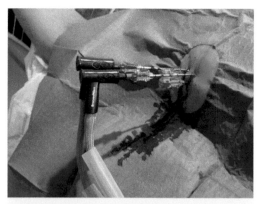

Fig. 3.191 Retracted coaxial needle with active antennas, tips still in skin entry level. Two remaining coaxial needles also still in place.

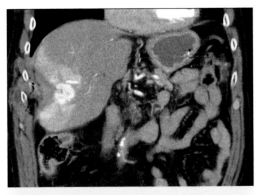

Fig. 3.192 Coaxial reconstruction of contrast-enhanced CT shows thermal damage to the periphery of the right liver lobe and the abdominal wall. The tumor nodule is vividly taking up contrast medium, ablation of the metastasis is not sufficient.

What Would You Do?

Notes:

_____

_____

_____

_____

_____

_____

_____

_____

Possible Strategies for Complication Management

- Operative reconstruction and tumor resection.
- Conservative treatment.
- Antibiosis.

Final Complication Management

A 3 cm skin necrosis developed and there was fistulation present, both of which were treated conservatively. Secondary healing of the skin defect occurred but lasted 5 months. The metastasis showed no further growth during this time but—from an oncologic standpoint—was not sufficiently treated (► Fig. 3.193a, b).

After the skin wound healed, a second ablation was scheduled. This time it was performed successfully with one antenna placed subsequently in different locations of the tumor. For each ablation run a direct puncture was used. This time the metastasis was treated sufficiently (► Fig. 3.194a, b). The patient is in complete remission 15 months following this procedure.

Complication Analysis

There are two possible reasons for this complication. First, there might have been transmission of heat to the abdominal wall through the two unused coaxial needles left in place (back heating), and second, there could have been unnoticed peripheral dislocation of one or both of the active antennas during ablation. This complication highlights the fact that extreme care must be taken when using MWA with coaxial guiding needles.

Strategies to Prevent and Take-Home Message

A coaxial MWA technique is cumbersome and potentially yields severe complications.

CT fluoroscopy should be considered to check for signs of dislocation or nontarget ablation especially during longer ablation runs.

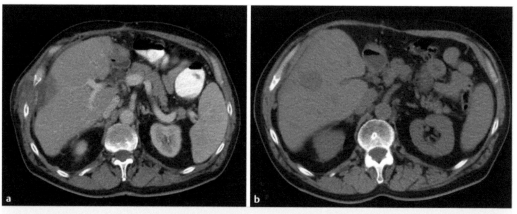

Fig. 3.193 **(a)** Residual Thickening of the abdominal wall 5 months after thermal damage from microwave ablation. **(b)** Five months after treatment the metastasis in the right liver lobe still present.

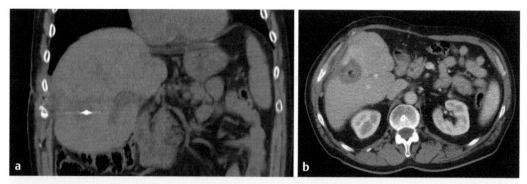

Fig. 3.194 **(a)** The tip of the microwave ablation (MWA) antenna located in the nodule. **(b)** Total tumor necrosis with safety margin following MWA.

Further Reading

Filippiadis DK, Tutton S, Mazioti A, Kelekis A. Percutaneous image-guided ablation of bone and soft tissue tumours: a review of available techniques and protective measures. Insights Imaging. 2014; 5(3):339–346

Liang P, Wang Y, Yu X, Dong B. Malignant liver tumors: treatment with percutaneous microwave ablation—complications among cohort of 1136 patients. Radiology. 2009; 251(3):933–940

Vogl TJ, Nour-Eldin NA, Hammerstingl RM, Panahi B, Naguib NNN. Microwave ablation (MWA): basics, technique and results in primary and metastatic liver neoplasms—review article. RoFo Fortschr Geb Rontgenstr Nuklearmed. 2017; 189(11):1055–1066

Kitchin D, Lubner M, Ziemlewicz T, et al. Microwave ablation of malignant hepatic tumours: intraperitoneal fluid instillation prevents collateral damage and allows more aggressive case selection. Int J Hyperthermia. 2014; 30(5):299–305

Yu H, Burke CT. Comparison of percutaneous ablation technologies in the treatment of malignant liver tumors. Semin Intervent Radiol. 2014; 31(2):129–137

Poggi G, Montagna B, DI Cesare P, et al. Microwave ablation of hepatocellular carcinoma using a new percutaneous device: preliminary results. Anticancer Res. 2013; 33(3):1221–1227

Index

Note: Page numbers set **bold** or *italic* indicate headings or figures, respectively.